Toxic Free

ALSO BY DEBRA LYNN DADD

1984   *Nontoxic & Natural*

1986   *The Nontoxic Home*

1990   *Nontoxic, Natural & Earthwise*
(in collaboration with Steve Lett and Judy Collins)

1992   *The Nontoxic Home & Office*

1997   *Home Safe Home*

2004   *Home Safe Home* (revised edition)

Toxic Free

How to Protect Your Health and Home from the Chemicals That Are Making You Sick

DEBRA LYNN DADD

JEREMY P. TARCHER/PENGUIN
a member of Penguin Group (USA) Inc.
New York

JEREMY P. TARCHER/PENGUIN
Published by the Penguin Group
Penguin Group (USA) Inc., 375 Hudson Street, New York, New York 10014, USA •
Penguin Group (Canada), 90 Eglinton Avenue East, Suite 700, Toronto, Ontario M4P 2Y3,
Canada (a division of Pearson Penguin Canada Inc.) • Penguin Books Ltd,
80 Strand, London WC2R 0RL, England • Penguin Ireland, 25 St Stephen's Green,
Dublin 2, Ireland (a division of Penguin Books Ltd) • Penguin Group (Australia),
250 Camberwell Road, Camberwell, Victoria 3124, Australia (a division of Pearson
Australia Group Pty Ltd) • Penguin Books India Pvt Ltd, 11 Community Centre,
Panchsheel Park, New Delhi–110 017, India • Penguin Group (NZ), 67 Apollo Drive,
Rosedale, North Shore 0632, New Zealand (a division of Pearson New Zealand Ltd) •
Penguin Books (South Africa) (Pty) Ltd, 24 Sturdee Avenue, Rosebank,
Johannesburg 2196, South Africa

Penguin Books Ltd, Registered Offices: 80 Strand, London WC2R 0RL, England

Portions of this book appeared in slightly different form in *Home Safe Home* (Tarcher/Penguin).
Copyright © 1997 by Debra Lynn Dadd

Most Tarcher/Penguin books are available at special quantity discounts for bulk purchase for sales
promotions, premiums, fund-raising, and educational needs. Special books or book excerpts also can
be created to fit specific needs. For details, write Penguin Group (USA) Inc. Special Markets,
375 Hudson Street, New York, NY 10014.

Library of Congress Cataloging-in-Publication Data

Dadd, Debra Lynn, date.
Toxic free : how to protect your health and home from the chemicals that are making you sick /
Debra Lynn Dadd.
p.   cm.
Includes bibliographical references and index.
ISBN 978-1-58542-870-0 (pbk.)
1. Household supplies—Toxicology—Popular works.   2. Product safety—Popular works.   3. Consumer
education—Popular works.   4. Housekeeping—Popular works.   5. Substitute products—Popular works.
I. Title.
RA1213.D336   2011   2011019687
363.19—dc23

Printed in the United States of America
1   3   5   7   9   10   8   6   4   2

Neither the publisher nor the author is eng█████ ██ ██████ ███████ █l advice or services to the individual
reader. The ideas, procedures, and sugges█████ contained in this book are not intended as a substitute for
consulting with your physician. All matters regarding your health require medical supervision. Neither the
author nor the publisher shall be liable or responsible for any loss or damage allegedly arising from any
information or suggestion in this book.

While the author has made every effort to provide accurate telephone numbers and Internet addresses at the
time of publication, neither the publisher nor the author assumes any responsibility for errors, or for changes
that occur after publication. Further, the publisher does not have any control over and does not assume any
responsibility for author or third-party websites or their content.

For

Larry Redalia

Thank you for twenty-four
years of helping me be
toxic-free.

Good,
the more Communicated,
more abundant grows.

—JOHN MILTON, *Paradise Lost*

ACKNOWLEDGMENTS

THIS BOOK is the current incarnation of a book that was first published in 1984 and has been continuously in print in one version or another for more than two decades. Over the years, many people have contributed to this book being what it is today.

I want to thank Jeremy P. Tarcher for taking a chance with me as a first-time author, and Joel Fotinos, publisher of Tarcher, for continuing to publish each new book when Tarcher became an imprint of Penguin.

I would also like to thank my editor, Michael Solana, who was delightful to work with and made a valuable contribution to the organization of material in this book, and my copy editor, David Chesanow.

My literary agent, Jay Poynor, has been a joy.

Especially I want to acknowledge Dr. Steven Lund, DC, LMT, for reviewing the portions of this book regarding physiology and detoxification. His extensive knowledge and experience in this area were of great assistance to me, and I feel confident that everything I have written is correct.

And in particular I want to acknowledge all the businesses that make and sell toxic-free products. You make it possible for us to choose health.

CONTENTS

CHAPTER 3 Environment 111

CHAPTER 4 Body 129

AUTHOR'S NOTE

SPEAK TO YOU not as a doctor, scientist, or toxicologist, but as an educated consumer. Just like you, I want to create a home that is comfortable, enjoyable, and safe. Think of me like a friend or neighbor, sharing homemaking tips across the fence or over a cup of tea.

You can also consider me to be a mentor—an experienced and knowledgeable adviser who can show you the way to do something, in a field that can be confusing and overwhelming. By allowing me to guide you through unfamiliar territory, you will be able to learn more quickly and easily for yourself how to make your own decisions regarding toxic chemicals.

This book contains information I have gathered regarding choices you can make that can improve your health. I am not a medical doctor and I am not giving you medical advice. The information in this book has not been evaluated by the FDA. Nothing in this book is intended to diagnose, treat, cure, or prevent any disease, disorder, pain, injury, deformity, or physical or mental condition. Individual results may vary.

In this book I am simply sharing with you knowledge I have gained from extensive research and personal experience, which has helped me and others I know improve our health. I believe that if you apply the information in this book in your own life, you can improve your health, too, but to do so is entirely your choice and the consequences of doing so, or not, are entirely your responsibility.

Occasionally in this book I make suggestions for using products in ways other than those for which they were originally intended. Because government regulations do not allow manufacturers to recommend their products for certain uses without laboratory proof that they are indeed safe and effective for such uses (and because they must procure government approval of the test results), these alternative uses are not necessarily approved by the manufacturer. Not all the suggestions given are guaranteed to work for everyone, but all have been found to work for many people.

This book is designed to serve people with different interests, budgets, medical conditions, and lifestyles, and as such it may occasionally make recommendations that are not appropriate for you. At these times, simply make an individual choice, and remember that the book's primary purpose is to make you aware of the toxic dangers in your home and the environment and suggest toxic-free alternatives.

Because your body is unique, you alone must make the decisions regarding how you take care of it. My intent in writing this book is simply to offer you information that will help you in your own choice to be toxic-free.

toxic

- the damage caused by a poison

free

- not under the control or in the power of another; able to act or be done as one wishes without hindrance or restraint
  - not subject to domination
  - not being imprisoned or enslaved
- not physically restrained, obstructed, or impeded
- (**free from**) not being subject to or affected by (a particular undesirable thing)
- (**-free**) not containing a specified substance
- having the power of self-determination—the ability to make one's own decisions, act independently of circumstances, and dictate one's own future

toxic-free

- an object—such as a product, a home, or a body—that does not contain toxic chemicals
- free from exposure to toxic chemicals
- free from contamination with toxic chemicals
- free from the harmful effects of toxic chemicals to body, mind, and spirit
- free from the oppression of toxic chemicals and able to manage the risks associated with them
- having the intent to be healthy, even while living in a toxic world

Introduction

Within each of us is an immeasurable capacity for love, understanding, compassion, creativity, joy, and all positive qualities. The tragedy of illness is that it prevents the full expression of outgoing healthy emotions and creative abilities. . . .

I feel that the achievement of health is worth considerable effort and expense because it can add happiness to our lives and to others, can help us to know love and warmth, song, laughter, and music, to experience the joy of creativity and the satisfaction of accomplishments well done.

—ADELE DAVIS

Let's Get Well (1972 ed.)

F YOU ARE READING THIS BOOK, it is likely you have toxic chemicals in your body that are making you sick.

That's a bold statement, I know, but throughout this book I will show you the truth of it.

I will also tell you how you can reduce the toxic chemical load in your body and how you can remove the consumer products that are making your home toxic, so that you and your loved ones can enjoy the good health that is your birthright.

I have been living without toxic chemicals in my home for more than thirty years. Creating a toxic-free home changed my life:

- I recovered my health.
- I save money on health care costs.
- I enjoy life more because my body feels good: I can work and have fun.

It was my father, actually, who first introduced me to the idea that toxic chemicals might be making me sick.

When I was twenty-four, I moved back home from living on my own to take care of my mother, who was dying of cancer. She had tried many treatments, but now the doctors told her that her time was short, and I moved back to my parents' house to take care of her during her last days. She lived only another month. She was only fifty-one. Both my grandmothers also died of cancer. When I began to write this book, two of my friends were battling breast cancer, and one died before I finished.

One night, shortly after my mother died, I was sitting at the piano, playing a very beautiful and moving piece of music that could bring tears to anyone's eyes, but I started crying uncontrollably. I just couldn't stop crying.

Now, I had plenty of reason to cry, but my father saw it differently. While my mother was living, he had wanted her to have intravenous vitamin C treatments. The hospital wouldn't administer the treatments, so he found a doctor who would. The doctor was one of the first to practice what is now called environmental medicine. While waiting for my mother to get her vitamin C, my father learned that one of the symptoms associated with toxic chemical exposure was hysterical crying. I went and got tested and was diagnosed with an immune system dysfunction caused by exposure to toxic chemicals, known then as environmental illness and now called multiple chemical sensitivities or MCS.

It wasn't any disease that I could recognize. Hysterical crying was only part of it. I had a whole set of symptoms that seemed totally unrelated. At my worst, I had constant headaches and insomnia every night. Taking a shower made me feel faint, and most of the time I couldn't think clearly. I had strong, sudden uncontrollable urges to eat anything and everything that had sugar in it—a carton of ice cream, a box of cookies, a whole coconut cream pie—and I usually was very depressed.

I couldn't go anywhere because there were toxic chemicals everywhere that would make me sick. I had a diagnosis but no treatment. I knew toxic chemicals were making me sick, but I didn't know what to do to get well.

About a year later, having not improved at all, another woman with MCS asked me, "Are you still sleeping on permanent-press sheets? They have a lot of formaldehyde on them, you know." This question changed my life. It actually had never occurred to me there were toxic chemicals *in my home* that were making me sick. Wasn't the government watching out for things like that? Apparently not.

This was the first time anyone had suggested to me that I find out where the toxic chemicals were in my home that were making me sick. And so I did.

When I first started studying toxic chemicals and their health effects in 1978, there was not a lot of information. I had to dig up whatever I could find from poison control centers, medical libraries, and toxicology books. There were no indoor-air-quality studies or nonprofit organizations devoted to researching toxics, or household hazardous-waste collection programs (we didn't even know then that there *was* household hazardous waste). And the results of toxic chemical studies certainly weren't in the news almost every day as they are today. It was like playing detective. My quest to find where toxic chemicals were hidden in my home was what got me out of bed every morning. I wanted to know what was making me sick so I could get well.

Day by day I began to associate particular symptoms with specific exposures. When I put on perfume, immediately I would get a headache; when I stopped wearing perfume, my headaches stopped.

Because I felt faint in the shower, I asked my father to rig up a filter that would remove chlorine; when he installed it, I no longer felt faint when I showered. After reading that formaldehyde caused insomnia and that formaldehyde was in the permanent-press finish on bedsheets, I changed my sheets to pure wrinkled cotton and could finally sleep.

As I learned more and more about where toxic chemicals were hidden in consumer products I was using every day, it began to seem like *everything* in my house was toxic—and, in fact, it was.

One day I decided I needed to get *all* the toxic chemicals out of my house. And I did. Like a tornado, all in one day, I swept through and removed all the products that contained toxic chemicals from my home. When I was done, all that was left was four bare walls, a concrete floor with dried paint spatters all over it (which had previously been covered by carpet), and a metal roll-away bed frame with a pile of cotton thermal blankets for a mattress.

But there were no toxic chemicals in the room.

And my body began to heal.

When I saw that exposure to toxic chemicals in the consumer products I used in my home had made me sick, and that I could improve my health by avoiding them, I could see that this entire ordeal I had gone through with my health *could have been prevented.*

I didn't want anyone else to needlessly get sick because they didn't know they were being exposed to toxic chemicals right in their own homes. And so I started writing about toxic chemicals in the home, and safe alternatives to those chemicals.

I started with a little book that I self-published by making photocopies. And doors started to open. The makers of Bon Ami Polishing Cleanser sent me on two national media tours because I was recommending Bon Ami as a nontoxic product.

Then I met a book editor and wrote my first real book, *Nontoxic & Natural,* which was published in 1984. In 1986, I wrote *The Nontoxic Home,* a primer for identifying household toxics and getting started with making changes. Both *Nontoxic & Natural* and *The Nontoxic Home* were updated in the early 1990s to *Nontoxic, Natural & Earthwise* and *The Nontoxic Home & Office.* In 1997 they were combined into *Home Safe Home,* which was rereleased in a revised edition in 2004. As I write today, my books on household toxics and safe alternatives have been continuously in print with the same publisher for more than twenty-five years.

Three significant things have happened since I wrote my last book:

- Many more nontoxic and natural products have been introduced into the marketplace.

- Much more information has become available on the health effects of toxic chemicals found in consumer products.
- Legislation is being introduced at both federal and state levels to strengthen the laws that govern toxic chemicals in consumer products.

Practically every week now, there is a new study in the news about toxic chemicals in consumer products and how they can make us sick.

There is no longer any question that there are toxic chemicals in consumer products or that they affect our health. The question we are faced with today is: What can we do to protect our health from all these toxic chemicals?

The answers are here in this book.

There is now so much information about household toxics and safe alternatives that I am not even going to attempt to be comprehensive.

Instead, I am going to open a door to a new world for you to explore with a "quick-start" guide. My aim with this book is to give you, in easy-to-understand language:

- a basic understanding of how toxic chemicals in consumer products can affect your health
- easy first steps that anyone can do to remove toxic exposures from your home
- tips on how you can reduce the amount of toxic pollution you put into the environment
- tools you can use to help your body detox and recover from the toxic burden it already has

There are many reasons why you might choose to be toxic-free.

The most obvious, of course, is that it is better for your health. We now know that exposure to toxic chemicals can contribute to virtually every illness (more about that in Chapter 1).

But you can also save money on medical bills. A report released in 2010 by the Safer Chemicals, Healthy Families coalition (www.safer chemicals.org) estimates that $5 billion would be saved on health care costs in America each year if we eliminated toxic chemicals in consumer products that translated into only one-tenth of one percent of health care costs. Some 133 million people in the United States—almost half of all Americans—have some sort of chronic disease or condition related to toxic chemical exposures. Seventy percent of deaths and 75 percent of U.S. health care costs are now attributed to toxic chemicals in consumer products we use in our homes every day.

Many of the consumer products we use at home can also affect the environment, releasing toxic substances either in their manufacture, use, or disposal. A large majority of the products that are toxic to humans are synthesized from petrochemicals, which cause pollution ranging from oil spills to toxic waste, to which we are then exposed through air pollution, water pollution, and food grown in contaminated soil.

But while finishing up the writing of this book, I learned something more that made me realize how urgent it is right now to address the problem of toxics in consumer products.

I was reading a book called *Radical Medicine: Cutting-Edge Natural Therapies That Treat the Root Causes of Disease* by Dr. Louisa L. Williams. I met her in 2008 when I was speaking at the Weston Price Foundation conference in San Francisco. She knew exactly who I was, as she had read my books. Dr. Williams was delighted to meet me and gave me a copy of her five-pound, three-inch-thick book, in which she had cited one of my books as a reference. I noted her book was about treating illness as a result of toxic chemical exposure, brought the book home, and put it on a shelf to read as soon as I had time.

Finally, on Winter Solstice 2010, I opened the book, and on the very first page Dr. Williams said:

> An apple a day won't keep the doctor away . . . nor can the most optimum diet possible, drinking pure water, exercising regularly or even diligently supplementing with mega-doses of vitamins and minerals ensure the preservation of good health for most Americans. *A healthy lifestyle [is] simply no longer adequate to fend off degenerative disease and help individuals regain their birthright of optimal health.* (italics mine)

Dr. Williams went on to say that such natural practices as chiropractic and other natural remedies are no longer as effective as they were one hundred years ago, before our bodies began to be inundated with toxic chemicals. I asked a friend of mine who is a chiropractor about this and he said yes, this is true, many chiropractors are now offering other services, such as nutrition, because at times classic chiropractic does not work as it did when it was first developed in 1895.

I was stunned to read this. Since 1987 my basic truth has been if I just follow nature's ways, all will be well. It is not just that we should all be eating whole foods, drinking eight glasses of water every day, taking vitamins, exercising, getting enough sleep, and availing ourselves of the many natural remedies available; it's that, alone, these commonsense health guidelines are not enough to handle the onslaught of toxic chemicals we are daily exposed to in our homes and the environment, and the toxic chemicals that are already stored in our bodies from past exposures.

We can't even lose weight by dieting alone anymore, as Suzanne Somers pointed out in her newest book, *Sexy Forever: How to Fight Fat After Forty*. The first step in her new weight-loss program is to reduce your toxic exposures and detox stored toxic chemicals from your body. Then a correct diet will work.

Our human bodies now have a new condition that wasn't in the original plan: toxic overload. We no longer live in a world where our bodies can be healthy solely as a result of a healthy lifestyle. We need to address our toxic exposure first. Every decision now needs to be made around the question: Does this action contribute to or reduce toxic exposure to individual humans or the environment?

As depressing as this might sound, learning that we are at a point where our bodies now may be too toxic to be healed by natural means only gave me the determination to do so. The fact is there are many things we can do to detox our bodies and clean up our homes and the environment. It became clear to me that NOW is the time to do them. And do them big-time. Everyone. Everywhere. We've hit bottom. Now it's time to come up.

Today it is easier than ever to replace toxic products in your home with safe ones, and there are gentle—yet effective—detox methods to remove toxic chemicals from your body, one of which is as simple as placing a few drops of flavorless liquid in a glass of water.

All you need to do to reverse the harmful effects of toxic chemicals on your health is choose to be toxic-free, learn what to do, and do it.

CHAPTER 1

Toxics

An error doesn't become a mistake until you refuse to correct it.

—ORLANDO A. BATTISTA, award-winning chemist

XPOSURE TO toxic chemicals can make you sick, but the sickness toxic chemicals cause is not an illness, like an infection caused by bacteria or viruses that can be treated by taking a drug. Rather, the sickness that results from toxic chemical exposure is a condition—a state of impaired working order that can be reversed by removing the toxic exposure that caused it, just as the condition of sunburn will heal when you stay out of the sun. It's something we have a choice over and can do something to prevent.

I expect exposure to toxic chemicals in the consumer products we use every day will soon be recognized as the number one health issue in the world today. Given the widespread use of toxic chemicals in consumer products and the prevalence of toxics throughout the environment, the subject of toxics is one everyone needs to know about.

By the time you finish reading this book, I want you to feel confident that you can choose to be toxic-free and know how to protect your health from the potentially devastating effects of toxic chemical exposure.

To every subject there are basic fundamentals. If you understand these basic concepts, you can then understand anything you read or hear about toxic chemicals and evaluate the dangers for yourself. You can free yourself from the opinions of others and find out for yourself what is true.

Knowing about toxic chemicals, how they can affect your health, and how to protect yourself and your loved ones from toxic exposure is an extremely useful subject in the world today because we encounter toxic exposures all around us as we go about our lives. Having this knowledge could mean the difference between enjoying a healthy, happy life making your dreams come true and a life of pain, suffering, and astronomical medical expenses. If you care about your health and the health of your loved ones, you need this information.

There is a whole field called toxicology that addresses how toxic chemicals affect your body (I've explained the basics of this field in Appendix B in the back of this book). For the moment, though, there are four key points to understand about toxics.

Toxics Are Poisons

A *poison* is a substance that can, in sufficient quantity, injure or kill a body. Some well-recognized poisons include arsenic, cyanide, and mercury. Until about two hundred years ago, there was only one kind of poison, the kind that appears in nature:

Microbial poisons are produced by bacteria and fungi. Botulinum toxin, for example, is produced by the bacterium *Clostridium botulinum* and is capable of inducing weakness and paralysis when underprocessed, non-acidic canned foods or other foods containing the spores are eaten.

Plant poisons are found in many plants, both wild and domesticated. Even some common plants we know and love contain poisons, such as daffodils, irises, tulips, and some chrysanthemums. The eyes of potatoes contain poisons and should not be eaten.

Animal poisons are usually transferred through the bites and stings of venomous animals. On land, this includes poisonous snakes, scorpions, spiders, and ants; in water, sea snakes, stingrays, and jellyfish.

Smoke contains poisons in the form of combustion by-products, including formaldehyde, nitrogen dioxide, sulfur dioxide, carbon dioxide, and hydrogen cyanide. These chemicals are released during the burning of wood in forest fires and the eruption of volcanoes.

At the beginning of the 1800s, however, the Industrial Revolution brought many changes to the world, among them large-scale production of chemicals. These new methods resulted in the creation of two new types of poisons that had never before been introduced into the living world.

REFINED CHEMICALS

Refined chemicals are made by separating a whole natural substance into its component parts.

An example of this is the making of sodium chloride. In nature, salt is found in bodies of salt water and in underground mines that once were salty seas. This salt is composed of sodium and chloride plus all the minerals and trace elements that exist in nature. This whole, natural salt was the salt that was eaten by everyone since the beginning of time, until the Industrial Revolution.

When industrial processes were developed, salt was refined, separating out the pure sodium chloride needed for industrial processes from the "impurities" (minerals and trace elements). Today the word *salt* means "refined industrial sodium chloride." You need to buy sea salt or mined Himalayan salt or one of the other specialty salts to get whole salt as it exists in nature.

MAN-MADE CHEMICALS

Once whole natural substances were refined into their component parts, industry took these substances—particularly refined crude oil—and made new chemicals that don't exist in nature.

An example of this is the making of pesticides. Almost all pesticides are made from hydrocarbons derived from petroleum. Before pesticides can be made, crude oil must be removed from the earth using oil derricks and wells, and that crude oil must be shipped to a refinery, where the crude oil is distilled into various substances, including petroleum. Other refined industrial chemicals are added, such as chlorine, sulfur, phosphorus, and nitrogen. Liquid pesticides use a mix of whatever petroleum distillates are available at the time of manufacture as "inert ingredients."

Today, most of the poisons we are exposed to are refined and man-made synthetic chemicals, found in consumer products we use every day.

I found it interesting that some substances we think of as poisons are not, in fact, poisonous in their natural state, only in their industrialized form.

It is widely known, for example, that the refined sodium chloride we call salt is one of the risk factors that contribute to high blood pressure, which substantially increases the risk of developing heart disease or stroke. On the other hand, whole natural salt, with its full spectrum of minerals, has a long list of benefits, including regulating blood pressure, maintaining electrolyte levels, and improving the immune system.

Another example is chromium. Chromium is one of the basic elements found on the periodic table of the elements. It is mined from nature as chromite ore. The toxicity of chromium varies according to its form. Trivalent chromium is actually required by our bodies in trace amounts for sugar metabolism (diabetics take it as a dietary supplement to lower blood sugar) and its deficiency may cause a disease called chromium deficiency. However, hexavalent chromium (the chemical of concern in the movie *Erin Brockovich*) is very toxic and damages DNA in your cells when inhaled.

Nowadays, most consumer products are made from petrochemical derivatives of nonrenewable crude oil. Often these compounds are not otherwise found in nature, and our bodies have not developed the means to identify or assimilate them. These chemicals are used in nearly every industry and every type of consumer product.

The adjective *toxic* refers to the damage caused by a poison. It is used to describe both the poison itself having the ability to damage as well as the body that has been damaged.

Toxic comes from the Greek word *toxon*, which means "bow," as in bow and arrow. The Greek term *toxikon pharmakon* means "poison arrows" made with the natural poison from the poison dart frog. These were used in hunting, the poison being an aid to killing the animal. So something "toxic" has the character of a bow, being a weapon to kill things.

The noun *toxic* is a *man-made* toxic agent, a poison. These are also called *toxicants*. (Note that a *toxin* is a *naturally occurring* poisonous sub-stance that is a specific product of the metabolic activities of a living organism, notably toxic when introduced into the tissues, such as the botulinum toxin I mentioned earlier. Frequently this word is used incor-rectly to refer to a man-made poison when the word *toxic* or *toxicant* should have been used.)

To *intoxicate* is to have *man-made* poisons introduced from the out-side into one's body, especially in amounts that cause body functions to be impaired. Though this word also has the definitions of causing someone to lose control of their faculties or behavior, and to excite or exhilarate, and it is generally exclusively used in reference to alco-holic beverages, the original meaning of the word is "to put a poison into." And this applies to all poisons. We quite literally are intoxicated by toxic chemicals we are exposed to every day.

The *toxicity* of a poison is the relative degree of harm caused by it.

Toxicology is the science of poisons and their effects, particularly on living systems.

For there to be a poisoning, there must be four elements in place:

* a poison
* a body being exposed to the poison
* enough exposure to the poison that a toxic level of the chemical accumulates in the cells of the target tissue or organ
* a resultant injury to the cells that disrupts their normal structure or function, which is visible in signs and symptoms or death

IF THERE IS NO POISON, THERE IS NO POISONING

This may seem like an obvious statement to make; however, millions of people are suffering from health problems today and the environment is being destroyed because we don't recognize the poisons around us and eliminate them.

No poison—no poisoning. It's that simple.

There Are Tons of Toxics

There are, literally, tons of toxic chemicals in the world—in consumer products, in your home, in your child's school, in your workplace, in your community, and in the environment.

Once a year, in July, an industry publication called *Chemical & Engineering News* publishes statistics on industrial chemical production.

Here are the numbers for chemical production in the United States for 2009 (reported in July 2010).

Chemical Production in the United States in 2009	
organic chemicals	
(carbon-based compounds)	
such as acrylonitrile, benzene, styrene, urea, vinyl	72.5 million tons
inorganic chemicals	
(all chemicals that are not carbon-based)	
such as aluminum, ammonia, chlorine, sulfuric acid	77.3 million tons
plastics	
such as PET, styrene, PVC	32.2 million tons
synthetic fibers	
such as acrylic, nylon, polyester, rayon	2.5 million tons
synthetic fertilizers	65 million tons
TOTAL	248 million tons or 496 billion pounds

Source: *Chemical & Engineering News* 88(27), July 5, 2010

In 2009, the United States produced almost 500 billion pounds of chemicals and chemical products. This adds up to around 1,600 pounds of chemicals—about 10 times your body weight if you weigh 160 pounds—for each of the 310.9 million people in the United States.

All industrial chemicals must be registered with the Chemical Abstracts Service (www.cas.org), a division of the American Chemical Society. The Chemical Abstracts Services issues a CAS# (also called CASRN) for each chemical, which identifies it as a unique chemical. Because chemicals often have many common names and brand names, the CAS# gives the "official" identification, much like the scientific name of a plant or animal that has multiple common names. When you look up information on the health effects of chemicals to find out how toxic they are, you always want to check the CAS#.

More than 57 million CAS#s have been assigned to unique organic and inorganic chemicals. On the Chemical Abstracts Service website, there is a counter that changes every time a new CAS# is assigned. As I'm sitting here watching it today (November 15, 2010), the number is at 57,110,200, and counting. In the time it took me to type 57,110,200, it switched to 57,100,201.

Some of these chemicals are considered safe for human use, but the vast majority have not been fully tested.

Almost no tests have been undertaken to evaluate the possible synergistic reactions that occur when chemicals are combined in food, water, or air, or when chemicals interact with other chemicals in our bodies. The few studies that have been done indicate that such combinations increase risks dramatically. Because scientists do not understand the ultimate effects of these chemicals, the government cannot begin to regulate their use sufficiently.

The average American home is literally filled with products made from these inadequately tested synthetic substances; we use more chemicals in our homes today than were found in a typical chemistry lab at the turn of the century. When professionals use chemicals in industrial settings, they are subject to strict health and safety codes, yet we use some of these same chemicals at home without guidance or restriction.

As further research is done, scientists are finding that many household products we assumed to be safe are actually toxic to some degree or another. A multitude of common symptoms such as headaches and depression can be related to exposure to household toxics. Insomnia, for example, is listed in toxicology books as a common symptom from exposure to the formaldehyde resin used on your bedsheets to keep them wrinkle-free. Yet, there is no regulation that requires this, or other health effects of formaldehyde, to be listed on the product label.

Bodies Collect and Store Toxic Chemicals

There is such a huge volume of toxic chemicals in the world today that there are far more than our bodies were designed to handle.

When your body's detox system is insufficient to remove the amount of toxic chemicals you are exposed to—and this applies to virtually everyone alive today—then the toxicants that come into your body will not be excreted, but instead will be stored in your body: in fat, semen, breast milk, muscles, bones, the brain, the liver, and other organs.

The total amount of these chemicals that are being stored in your body at a given point in time is called your *body burden*.

Various chemicals move through your body at different rates. Arsenic, for example, is mostly excreted within seventy-two hours of exposure. Some pesticides can remain in your body for fifty years.

Of course, how quickly chemicals are removed from your body depends on the condition of your body's detoxification system and the amount of toxic chemicals you are exposed to.

When you are continuously exposed to toxic chemicals—as most people are every day—more toxic chemicals enter the body than can be removed by your detoxification system, and body burden results.

Scientists say that everyone alive today is contaminated with at least seven hundred toxic chemicals in their bodies. It doesn't matter where you live or what you do. Just being on this planet, every body is contaminated.

EPA biopsies of human fat show:

- We all have polychlorinated biphenyls (PCBs) in our bodies, from adhesives, carbonless copy paper, dyes, fluorescent light ballasts, inks, paints, pesticides, plastics, and many other consumer products. No longer manufactured or widely used since 1977, PCBs are still widespread in the environment. Currently our most significant exposure is in fish.
- We all have styrene in our bodies from Styrofoam coffee cups and takeout food containers.
- We all have dichlorobenzene in our bodies from breathing fumes from air fresheners, mothballs, and toilet-deodorizer blocks.
- We all have xylene in our bodies from breathing gasoline, paint varnish, shellac, rust preventatives, permanent markers, and cigarette smoke.
- We all have dioxins in our bodies. The major sources of dioxin are in our diet. Since dioxin is fat-soluble, it bioaccumulates, climbing up the food chain. A North American eating a typical North American diet will receive 93 percent of their dioxin exposure from meat and dairy products (23 percent is from milk and dairy alone; other large sources of exposure are beef, fish, pork, poultry, and eggs). In fish, these toxicants bioaccumulate up the food chain so that dioxin levels in fish are 100,000 times that of the surrounding environment.
- All these chemicals cause cancer as well as other illnesses.

All these chemicals and more are known to be stockpiled in everyone's bodies *unless you have done something to remove them*. (I'll discuss more about how you reduce your body burden by removing stored toxic chemicals in Chapter 4.)

Just how contaminated are our bodies in our current industrialized environment, compared to what it would be if the planet were not polluted with industrial chemicals?

An examination was done of lead in the bones of Peruvians buried

1,600 years ago. The Peruvian bones were compared to lead found in the bones of present-day residents of the United Kingdom and the United States. The amount of lead in the bones of present day human bodies is 1,000 times the amount found in the bones of ancient Peruvians.

That your body stores toxic chemicals is a good thing, because it keeps the chemicals from circulating through your body in your bloodstream and creating toxic effects. However, it's better to not hold on to those toxicants.

Your body has the ability to alter toxic chemicals to increase or decrease—or totally change—their effects. What makes toxic effects so unpredictable is that chemicals inside your body can react with other chemicals that enter your body at the same time, or that have already entered and been stored. A well-known example is alcoholic beverages and tranquilizers, but reactions can also occur between a cleaning product and a pesticide or even something as seemingly insignificant as a food additive. Carrying around past toxic exposures in your body, which can be released at any time, just increases your chances of toxic health problems.

Since 2001, the National Center for Environmental Health (NCEH) at the Centers for Disease Control and Prevention (CDC) has produced four reports called the *National Report on Human Exposure to Environmental Chemicals* (www.cdc.gov/exposurereport). These are a series of ongoing assessments of the U.S. population's exposure to environmental chemicals by measuring chemicals in a person's blood or urine, a process called biomonitoring. Biomonitoring results help CDC scientists find out what chemicals enter a person's body and at what concentration. The results also help scientists learn about the general population's exposure to certain chemicals.

The *Fourth National Report on Human Exposure to Environmental Chemicals 2009* is the most comprehensive assessment to date of the exposure of the U.S. population to chemicals in our environment. Some 212 chemicals were found in about 2,400 people tested.

The report's Executive Summary gives these findings regarding chemicals found in the bodies of Americans:

Polybrominated diphenyl ethers are fire retardants used in certain manufactured products. These accumulate in the environment and in human fat tissue. One type of polybrominated diphenyl ether, BDE-47, was found in the serum of nearly all of the NHANES participants.

Bisphenol A (BPA), a component of epoxy resins and polycarbonates, may have potential reproductive toxicity. General population exposure to BPA may occur through ingestion of foods in contact with BPA-containing materials. CDC scientists found bisphenol A in more than 90% of the urine samples representative of the U.S. population.

Another example of widespread human exposure included several of the perfluorinated chemicals. One of these chemicals, perfluorooctanoic acid (PFOA), was a byproduct of the synthesis of other perfluorinated chemicals and was a synthesis aid in the manufacture of a commonly used polymer, polytetrafluoroethylene, which is used to create heat-resistant non-stick coatings in cookware. Most participants had measurable levels of this environmental contaminant.

It is bad enough that these chemicals each individually are known to be hazardous to health. What is worse is that the dangers of exposure to these chemicals *in combination* has never been studied.

Toxics Contribute to Every Illness

Do you know someone who has been poisoned?

How about someone who currently has cancer or has died of cancer?

Do you know a couple that has not been able to conceive a child?

Anyone with diabetes or who is overweight?

How about anyone with chronic headaches or insomnia?

All of these conditions—and more—can be the result of exposure to toxic industrial chemicals.

Chances are, not only do you know people who have been made sick by toxic chemicals, but you yourself are suffering to some degree from exposure to toxic chemicals.

When I started researching toxic chemicals in consumer products we use at home in 1978, the field of toxicology barely existed. The first toxicology textbook wasn't written until 1971, and the first professional organization to certify toxicologists wasn't formed until 1979.

Today, more than a quarter of a century later, our knowledge of toxic chemicals and their health effects have changed dramatically. Studies now exist that show *toxic chemical exposure underlies virtually every symptom and illness.*

Two excellent websites to visit to find these studies are:

- Scorecard (www.scorecard.org/health-effects/index.tcl)
- The Collaborative on Health and the Environment (www.healthand environment.org/tddb/)

There is so much evidence that the toxic chemicals we encounter in our everyday exposures result in common diseases that I encourage all health care professionals—both conventional and alternative—to learn more about the associations between toxic exposures and illness, and to consider handling these exposures as a basic part of treatment.

In the health care world today, the primary focus is on symptoms. We experience a symptom, and then look for a remedy. Whether that remedy is a drug from a doctor or an herb from the natural-food store, we think in terms of finding a cure for signs and symptoms.

But there is another way to look at it. There are basic, core things that contribute to health, including adequate nutrition, exercise, sunlight, and other factors. When these life-supporting factors are present, the result is health. When they are not, illness results. Toxic chemical exposure is part of core wellness. When your body is exposed to toxicants, they can damage health throughout your body, and when you are free of these exposures, health happens; in fact, addressing toxic exposures nowadays is *necessary* for health to occur.

From my viewpoint, toxic chemicals are not just *a* major contributor to ill health, they are *the* major contributor to ill health. They are so widespread and cause such havoc in a body that toxic exposures should be among the first things considered and handled as part of creating a good foundation of health. Today, more and more health care professionals agree.

I am encouraged to see that over the thirty years during which I have been researching and writing on this subject, the trend is toward more and more awareness of how toxic exposures impact our health. We have the data. The associations have been made. We now need to integrate this knowledge into our health care practices.

But you don't need to wait for professional services or government regulations to reduce your exposure to toxic chemicals. You can yourself choose to be toxic-free. And you can encourage your own doctor and other health care professionals you see to learn more about how toxic exposures might be contributing to your own less-than-optimum or poor body conditions.

Poisons can affect every part of your body. For details on how toxic chemicals can affect each of your body systems, see Appendix A: How Toxics Affect Your Body Systems.

You Can Be Toxic-Free

The reason toxics are a health problem today is simple:

* We are exposed to too many toxic chemicals.
* Our bodies have too little capacity to eliminate the huge amounts of toxics we are exposed to.

To be healthy in today's toxic world, you need to:

* reduce the amount of your toxic exposures
* increase the ability of your body to process and eliminate toxic chemicals.

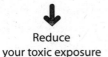
Reduce
your toxic exposure

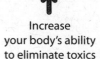
Increase
your body's ability
to eliminate toxics

You can do something about this.

You will find out how to reduce your exposure to toxic chemicals in consumer products you use at home in Chapter 2, and how to reduce your exposure to toxic chemicals in the environment in Chapter 3.

Then you will learn how to increase your body's ability to eliminate toxics in Chapter 4.

So read on. . . .

CHAPTER 2

Home

We shape our dwellings, and afterwards our dwellings shape us.

—WINSTON CHURCHILL

WHEN YOU move in to a new home, you start with empty rooms, which you can fill with whatever you want. And then you live in the environment you have created.

Since you have the power to place whatever you want in your home, you have the power to create a home environment that is toxic-free.

The most effective way to reduce your risk of getting sick from toxic chemical exposure is to simply avoid consumer products that contain toxic chemicals. Remember, if there is no poison present, there can be no poisoning.

While that may seem easier said than done, in fact, today it is entirely possible to remove virtually all major toxic chemicals from your home. I have lived in a toxic-free home since 1978; that's more than thirty years, so I know it can be done.

And it's much more enjoyable to live in a toxic-free home than a toxic one. There is no deprivation. It's much nicer to sleep on soft cotton sheets than scratchy polyester. Organically grown food is much more delicious, and nutritious. Natural essential oils have a lovelier fragrance in handmade soap. There's nothing not to like about living toxic-free.

Whether your home is a toxic place for you to live or not depends on:

- the toxic chemicals that are present in your home.
- the ability of your home to eliminate toxic chemicals, usually through ventilation.

The more toxic chemicals you have in your home, the more they build up into higher and higher concentrations if the windows are closed to conserve energy during winter heating or summer cooling. Here in Florida, we use air-conditioning about half of the year. If we had toxic chemicals in our home, the indoor air would get more and more toxic as the summer progresses, as air in heating, ventilation, and air-conditioning systems (HVAC) is recycled.

The Environmental Protection Agency (EPA) has established that our greatest exposure to toxic chemicals is right in our own homes. In 1987 they conducted an ambitious program to identify and compare the severity of various environmental problems, in the belief that in a world of limited resources, the agency should be focusing on those pollutants that pose greater dangers to society. The task force of agency managers and outside experts were surprised to find, right up at the top of the list: indoor air pollution from radon, space heaters, gas ranges, pesticides, and cleaning solvents, as well as pollutants evaporating from tap water—all of which we are exposed to at home.

So the place to begin with reducing your exposure to toxic chemicals is in your own home, where you have the greatest exposure and the greatest control.

It can seem like there are a lot of toxic chemicals you need to remove from your life, but in fact, the solutions are quite simple. Because choosing one toxic-free product can eliminate quite a number of toxic chemical exposures. Choosing fresh organic food, for example, eliminates pesticides, bisphenol A leaching from cans, plastic residues from packaging, and other toxic chemicals. Choosing not to wear perfume or use scented products with synthetic fragrances eliminates about four thousand toxic substances. Choosing natural-fiber clothing eliminates synthetic plastic fibers as well as formaldehyde-based fabric finishes.

In this chapter, you'll learn fifty simple, mostly inexpensive things you can do in your home to replace toxic products with products that are toxic-free, all around your home. Some cost nothing at all. They are grouped into these categories:

- The Big Five
- Indoor Air Pollution
- Household Cleaning and Laundry Products
- Household Pest Control
- Water
- Beauty and Hygiene
- Food
- Textiles
- Interior Decorating
- Home office

This is not a complete list of all toxic exposures in your home, but it covers most of the major exposures, and each is a good first step.

When I made the decision to remove toxic chemicals from my home, I just went on a rampage and removed all the toxic chemicals I knew about, all in one day. But you don't have to be that drastic.

As you read these recommendations, find *one* you think you can easily do. Start with that one. Do it, and congratulate yourself on a first step well taken. Then pick another one. Every time you take one step, you are reducing toxic exposures in your home and taking one step closer to good health.

And tell a family member or friend of your success. Encourage others you know to take that step. Even better, get together with some friends and do the steps together.

If you do all fifty, you will have made major progress toward making your home toxic-free.

I've put together a special page on my website with links to more information on how to implement each of these fifty steps, including recommended products and Q&A. Please visit www.debralynndadd.com/toxicfreebook-link.

And there is much more information on many more things you can do to eliminate toxic chemicals from your home on my website at www.debralynndadd.com.

Routes of Exposure

When assessing the risk of a product, it is very important to consider how the chemical is entering your body. Some substances do not give off fumes, but can be deadly if swallowed. Others may cause skin irritation and also cause reactions if they are inhaled. To help you quickly assess the danger, I have used four simple symbols to indicate the modes of exposure by which the product may be harmful. In many cases there are secondary exposures that are not recognized.

 Ingested by mouth

 Splashed in eyes

 Absorbed through the skin

 Inhaled through nose or mouth

For more information on routes of exposure, see Appendix B.
Toxic substances are set in **lowercase boldface type.**

The Big Five
Cigarette Smoke: First-, Second-, and Thirdhand

Surgeon General's Warning: Smoking causes lung cancer, heart disease, and emphysema, and may complicate pregnancy.

Surgeon General's Warning: Quitting smoking now greatly reduces serious risks to your health.

Surgeon General's Warning: Smoking by pregnant women may result in fetal injury, premature birth, and low birth weight.

Surgeon General's Warning: Cigarette smoke contains carbon monoxide.

TOBACCO SMOKE contains some of the most toxic air pollutants known, including **benzene, carbon monoxide, formaldehyde, ammonia, hydrogen cyanide**, and more than four thousand other chemicals—forty-three of which have been proven to cause cancer—and more than two hundred known poisons.

Even if you don't smoke but are around people who do on a regular basis, you can have similar health risks.

Cigarette smoke poses a hazard both to smokers and to nonsmokers as well. Only 4 percent of the total smoke produced by a cigarette is actually inhaled by the smoker. The other 96 percent becomes sidestream waste, containing more than twice the concentration of pollutants the smoker inhaled through the filter-tip. If you spend more than two hours in a room where someone is smoking, then you inhale toxicants equivalent to smoking four cigarettes.

In addition to putting thousands of toxic chemicals into your body, exposure to cigarette smoke destroys *cilia* in your lungs, impairing the ability of your lungs to clear inhaled particles. With each breath of cigarette smoke, you literally damage your lungs.

The EPA has designated secondhand smoke as a group A carcinogen.

In 2009, thirdhand smoke was identified as a possible risk for babies and children. Thirdhand smoke is tobacco smoke contamination that remains after the cigarette has been extinguished. The residual toxicants that linger in carpets and sofas, walls, and even the clothing and hair of smokers remain for hours and even days after a cigarette is put out. As of this writing, I couldn't find any studies directly linking thirdhand smoke to disease; however, that doesn't mean that it will not be found to be hazardous once studied. Thirdhand smoke can build up over time, especially on the walls of homes and cars where smokers have frequently smoked. I believe studies will find these places to be quite toxic.

HOW TO BE TOXIC-FREE

If you smoke, stop. At the very least, be considerate of nonsmokers and do not smoke in their immediate presence. A simple "Do you mind if I smoke?" will help you determine if you should step outside.

Don't allow anyone to smoke in your home, and support measures to make all public places smoke-free. Dangerous particles from cigarette smoke can remain in the air long after a cigarette has been extinguished.

If you live with a smoker, do everything you can to encourage him to quit, or ask her to smoke outside. Or you could designate a "smoking room." In Victorian times, men retired to a separate room and put on their "smoking jackets" before enjoying their tobacco, so as not to disturb the delicate constitutions of the women they lived with. But I don't think even this is sufficient. What's best for everyone's health and the environment is NO SMOKING.

Americans for Nonsmokers' Rights (www.no-smoke.org) has information on the science behind the risks of secondhand smoke and laws supporting smoke-free policies. You have a right to breathe smoke-free air, wherever you are.

I don't want to encourage smoking at all, but I do want to offer a "better than doing nothing" alternative for smokers: e-cigarettes. These battery-powered atomizers provide inhaled doses of tobacco-flavored nicotine by delivering a vaporized liquid nicotine solution to the lungs. When a smoker's body absorbs the nicotine, the smoker exhales a harmless water vapor that resembles smoke. This enables the smoker to get a nicotine fix anywhere without creating harmful secondhand smoke. Nicotine itself is a poison and I certainly am not saying it is not toxic. But if you are addicted to nicotine, or know someone who is, e-cigarettes eliminate all the extra exposure to the toxic chemicals in smoke, for yourself and others.

Alcoholic Beverages

ONE OR two drinks a day may not be harmful and, indeed, may be beneficial, but once this limit is passed, problems begin, and even this may be too much for some people.

Alcoholism can cause heart disease, hepatitis, cirrhosis of the liver, decreased resistance to disease, shortened life span, nutrient deficiencies, cancer, fetal alcohol syndrome, brain damage, stroke, phlebitis, varicose veins, and a reduced testosterone level in males, which can cause sexual impotence, loss of libido, breast enlargement, and loss of facial hair.

Unfortunately, the harmful effects of alcohol do not stop with the body of the drinker. Alcohol is responsible for many needless deaths caused by drunk drivers and is a factor in more than half of all the homicides, rapes, and sexually aggressive acts in this nation. Many alcoholics also die from falling, inability to escape during a fire, drowning, and suicide.

Another health concern about alcoholic beverages is that drinking alcohol can harm your liver, your body's most important detox organ. It also damages your nervous system, your cardiovascular system, and your immune system.

But most important to the subject of toxics risk is that even moderate alcohol consumption—just three days a week for several months—can lead to changes in how fast and by which pathways toxicants break down in your body. People who regularly drink alcoholic beverages are known to metabolize some chemicals faster than nondrinkers, which can increase the toxicity of these chemicals.

HOW TO BE TOXIC-FREE

I'm not going to tell you to never drink alcoholic beverages. I occasionally use wine or beer in cooking (which burns off the alcohol) and even more occasionally have a glass of wine or champagne on a special occasion.

The drinking of alcoholic beverages is one of those situations where you need to decide for yourself the amount and frequency of this poison that you are willing to risk, recognizing that it *is* a poison, and choosing what is appropriate for you.

That said, here are some guidelines for choosing beers and wines with the least amount of additional toxics.

Beer

Look for beers that use organically grown hops or malt. These are generally sold in natural-food stores.

A second choice would be natural beers. All German beers are protected by the Reinheitsgebot, or Purity Law, which makes it a crime to brew beer with ingredients other than hops, malt, and water. Also look for beers from small local breweries, which generally use the finest of natural ingredients, and because they are made in-house: you can ask all the questions you want to about what they are made from. Brewing beer at home also has become a popular pastime; if you want to try your hand at this, you can order supplies on the Internet.

Wine

Many natural-food stores sell very nice wines made from organically grown grapes. Some are imported from France, Germany, and Italy, quite a few are made in California, and wineries in other states also are going organic.

One major problem with wines, whether made from organically grown grapes or not, is the presence of sulfites, which can cause immediate breathing difficulties and other allergic reactions. Sulfites, generally considered food additives to be avoided, are formed naturally in the process of fermentation. Virtually all wines contain some sulfites; however, some winemakers also add sulfites to inhibit oxidation and spoilage, a practice that has been used for centuries. If a wine contains more than ten parts per million (ppm) sulfites, the statement "Contains sulfites" must appear on the label. Most wines contain 30 to 150 ppm.

If you wish to avoid alcoholic beverages entirely, a number of delicious nonalcoholic drinks are available at your natural-food store. Try one of the no-alcohol beers, a varietal grape juice made from wine grapes (I love these!), or a sparkling apple cider or other fruit juice instead of champagne.

Drugs

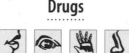

DRUGS FALL into three main categories: recreational, over-the-counter, and prescription. Recreational drugs are a subject unto themselves: their health effects are devastating and are best avoided altogether. Prescription drugs are best discussed with your medical doctor.

Here the subject is over-the-counter nonprescription drugs—painkillers, antacids, allergy medicines, cough syrups, laxatives, and sleeping pills—of the sort you might find in your medicine cabinet at home. It's a multibillion-dollar industry offering more than two thousand products.

An over-the-counter drug, as opposed to a prescription drug, is a drug product you can buy without a prescription and use when *you* think it is useful or necessary without a doctor's guidance. Over-the-counter drugs are formulated only to relieve symptoms and not to cure the underlying disease. They just make you less miserable so you can continue your daily routine while your body works on curing itself with its natural healing powers.

The biggest danger in having any kind of drug or medication in your home is the risk of accidental poisoning from an overdose. Children especially are attracted to the brightly colored pills and can quickly consume too many, with serious consequences.

Many drugs and medications have serious side effects, far too many to list here. To find out the side effects of the drugs in *your* medicine cabinet, go to your local library, where you can look up information on more than 2,500 popular pharmaceuticals in the *Physician's Desk Reference.* This is the standard reference that doctors use. You can also look up drugs online by simply typing the name of the drug into your favorite search engine.

In my opinion, the most harmful side effect of all drugs (recreational, over-the-counter, and prescription) is that many drugs can damage your liver, your most important detox organ. Most prescription drugs are man-made and cannot be assimilated by your body. These are stored in your body in the same manner as other toxic chemicals, thereby additionally contributing to your body's toxic overload.

Over-the-counter medications are meant to provide temporary relief for occasional symptoms, and are not to be used on a regular basis. As the label says, "If symptoms persist, see your doctor." You may have a more serious illness that requires medical attention.

HOW TO BE TOXIC-FREE

In previous books, I've given natural remedies you can make at home for relief of symptoms. But I've changed my viewpoint.

Symptoms are signals from your body that something is wrong and your body is doing something about it. When you run a fever, your body is heating up to kill germs; when you cough, it is clearing your lungs; a headache may be a sign that you are under too much stress and should take more leisure time for yourself. It's not always a good idea to stifle your symptoms, and never a good idea to ignore them completely, as they are part of your natural healing process.

Having attempted to heal my own symptoms for many years, without success, I decided to adopt a different strategy and heal my body "from the inside out"—that is, to address the underlying problems that are showing up as symptoms.

Changing my diet to not eat wheat handled a whole set of symptoms. Not eating refined white sugar handled others. Just going for a walk for twenty minutes a day around my neighborhood eliminated more symptoms. Drinking enough water took away still other symptoms.

But what I found to be most important of all was to remove the toxic chemicals from my body. I'll tell you more about this in Chapter 4.

Household Poisons and Hazardous Waste

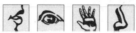

The most dangerous exposure your child has to household toxics is immediate poisoning from ingestion. According to the Centers for Disease Control and Prevention (CDC), in 2006, poison control centers reported about two million unintentional poisoning or poison exposure cases. Most poisonings involve everyday household items such as cleaning supplies, medicines, cosmetics, and personal care items.

Here are some real-life examples of how quickly a child can be poisoned. A one-year-old boy was watching his mother load the dishwasher. Without warning, he suddenly stuck his finger into the chlorinated dishwasher detergent and then put it in his mouth. A three-year-old died after drinking only three ounces of hair conditioner. Spilled laundry bleach caused the death of a baby after he crawled through it.

This risk is entirely eliminated when you simply don't have toxic products around the house.

A woman I know personally put down a spray bottle of all-purpose cleaner and went to answer the phone. Her two-year-old son grabbed it and sprayed it right into his eyes. Fortunately, it was a nontoxic cleaner, and he was fine.

If you are like I was, once you're convinced of the dangers of toxic products in your home, you're going to want to throw everything away and start using safe alternatives immediately! But when you do, you face the dilemma of proper disposal.

Why is disposal of household toxics a problem? Because when you dispose of your toxic household products, you generate what is called *household hazardous waste*. When you throw a half-used can of pesticide into the garbage, it will ultimately end up in a municipal landfill, which is designed for refuse, not toxic waste.

And most household poisons are also household hazardous waste.

Hazardous waste from households is not regulated like hazardous waste from industry and businesses are, even though the same toxic chemicals are involved.

The EPA estimates that 1 percent of all waste generated in the average American household is hazardous, with a national total of 1.6 million tons every year. The average home has accumulated as much as one hundred pounds of household hazardous waste that needs to be disposed of.

When household hazardous waste is not disposed of properly, it can be dangerous for sanitation workers and the environment. If household hazardous waste is dumped on the ground or poured into sewers, storm water can wash it into streams, lakes, and rivers, polluting drinking water sources. Household hazardous waste can also seep down through the ground until it reaches aquifers, which are underground sources of water, contaminating water sources for those who get their drinking water from wells. Plants and animals that live in or near the streams, lakes, and rivers can also be harmed from household hazardous waste in the water. Even household hazardous waste flushed down the toilet or poured into household drains simply goes through the municipal sewage-treatment plant before it is discharged into your local waterways.

HOW TO BE TOXIC-FREE

The very best thing you can do to reduce household poisonings and household hazardous waste is to simply stop using these dangerous products. You will be well on your way to doing so by following the fifty steps outlined in this book and the recommendations on my website (see Recommended Resources). You never have to buy products that might poison your children or pollute the environment again.

However, you are still faced with the problem of what to do with the household hazardous waste you already have. The answer is to take it to your local household hazardous-waste collection facility.

First, you need to *find* your local household hazardous-waste collection facility. I found mine by typing the name of my county and "household hazardous waste" into my favorite search engine online. I don't have any household hazardous waste to dispose of, but wanted to find out if my local community has a household hazardous-waste program. They do, and yours probably does too. If not, call the company that picks up your garbage and ask them what to do with your household hazardous waste. It may even be illegal to dispose of certain products with your normal household garbage.

Where I live, in Pinellas County, Florida, we have a location where we can drop off our household hazardous waste during normal business hours.

Every community has a list of what they will accept and what they won't accept, so get a list from your local disposal facility.

In general, though, here is a list of things to look for when identifying household poisons and hazardous waste in your home, from the San Francisco Household Hazardous Waste Program.

HOUSECLEANING SUPPLIES

Ammonia cleaners

Chlorine bleach

Cleansers

Disinfectants

Drain openers

Furniture and floor polish

Lye

Metal polish

Oven cleaner

Rug cleaners

Tub, tile, and shower-stall cleaners

Laundry supplies

Dry-cleaning solvent

Mothballs and flakes

Spot remover

COSMETICS

Cuticle remover

Depilatory cream

Hair—permanent wave solutions

Hair—straightening solutions

Nail polish

Nail polish remover

MEDICINES AND MEDICAL SUPPLIES

Chemotherapy drugs

Liquid medicine

Mercury from a broken thermometer

Prescription medicine

Rubbing alcohol

Lice shampoo

OTHER HOUSEHOLD PRODUCTS

Aerosol cans containing *any* pressure or fluid

Butane lighters

Lighter fluid

Shoe dye and polish

PET SUPPLIES

Flea powder

Pet shampoo

AUTOMOTIVE SUPPLIES

Aluminum cleaner

Auto-body filler

Automatic transmission fluid

Brake fluid

Carburetor cleaner

Car wax

Chrome polish

Diesel fuel

Engine degreaser

Gasoline

Kerosene or lamp oil

Lubricating oil

Motor oil, used (see if you can find a place that will accept this for recycling)

BUILDING AND WOODWORKING SUPPLIES

Asbestos

Fluorescent lamps with ballasts and tubes

Glues and cements

Wood preservatives

GARDEN SUPPLIES

Fungicides

Herbicides

Insecticides

Rat, mouse, and gopher poison

Snail and slug poison

Soil fumigants

Weed killers

HOBBY SUPPLIES

Acrylic paint

Artist's mediums, thinners, and fixatives

Chemistry sets

Oil paint

Photographic chemicals/solutions

Resins, fiberglass, and epoxy

Rubber cement thinner

Painting supplies

Latex-based paint

Model airplane paint

Oil-based paint

Paint stripper

Paint thinner, turpentine, and mineral spirits

Leave Toxics at the Door

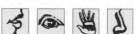

Even if you are careful to choose only nontoxic products to use in your home, every time you go outdoors you bring toxic chemicals back inside on the soles of your shoes. Chemicals can include asphalt, pesticides, and herbicides from lawns and gardens and sidewalks, and any number of other chemicals that may be present where you walk.

When you walk around your home with toxic chemicals on the soles of your shoes, they come off on the floor. Then, when you walk barefoot around your home, they can be absorbed through the soles of your feet. You can also inhale these chemicals as they vaporize. If you have children playing on the floor, the toxic chemicals can get on their hands and into their mouths. Children, especially infants, are even more susceptible to the dangers of toxic chemicals and carcinogens than adults.

HOW TO BE TOXIC-FREE

The solution is to leave your shoes at the door. Have a rack set up next to the door you enter most frequently, where you can leave your shoes when you enter the house. Have slippers or socks ready to put on if you don't want to go barefoot.

And remember to make provisions for guests and have slippers or socks available for them too.

Another thing to do is wash your hands first thing when you come indoors. As you walk around touching things, your hands can pick up toxic chemicals as well as germs.

One endocrine disruptor toxicant you are almost sure to pick up is bisphenol A (BPA), which is now found on many cash register receipts that use thermal paper. BPA transfers readily from receipts to skin and can penetrate the skin to such a depth that it cannot be washed off.

My grandmother used to always tell me to wash my hands after handling money because it was "filthy." She was right. Eighty-six percent of paper money tested at the Wright-Patterson Air Force Base's Wright-Patterson Medical Center carried germs that can be very dangerous to people whose immune systems are compromised, and with today's general exposure to immunotoxicants, this could be you. In addition, minute amounts of cocaine have been found on paper money, and 95 percent of dollar bills tested positive for BPA. What other untested toxics might also be on money?

Indoor Air Pollution
Air Filters

The reason for air filters is to remove pollutants from the air that are contributing to indoor air pollution.

Indoor air pollutants fall into three distinct categories:

Particulates: almost microscopic bits of material such as pollen, house dust, mold, animal dander, asbestos, and particles of tobacco smoke. If you need to remove particles from the air, you will probably know it because you'll have asthma or allergic symptoms such as sneezing, a runny nose, and itchy eyes.

Gases: misty vapors of volatile chemicals such as formaldehyde, plastics, paints, solvents, pesticides, perfumes, carbon monoxide, phenol, and tobacco-smoke gases. If you need to remove gases, you might have symptoms such as headache, fatigue, inability concentrating, or other symptoms of multiple chemical sensitivities.

Disease-causing organisms: bacteria and viruses.

THE EPA has called indoor air pollution the nation's number one environmental health problem. Since most people spend well over 90 percent of their time indoors, the quality of our indoor air impacts our health far more than that of outdoor air. According to the American College of Allergy, Asthma and Immunology, half of all illnesses are aggravated or caused by polluted indoor air. Fortunately, the quality of our indoor air is something each one of us can control.

Health effects from indoor air pollutants can be immediate or long-term. Immediate effects may show up after a single exposure or repeated exposures: irritation of the eyes, nose, and throat; headaches, dizziness, fatigue, and symptoms of asthma; hypersensitivity; and lung inflammation. Long-term effects include respiratory diseases, heart disease, and cancer, and can be severely debilitating or fatal. Because these long-term effects can take years to develop, it is prudent to improve the indoor air quality in your home even if you have no noticeable symptoms.

Indoor air pollution has become a problem because of the combination of sealing up homes for energy savings without appropriate ventilation equipment and then filling them with more and more toxic products. The level of toxic pollutants inside many homes is often higher than that of the air outside—sometimes even higher than the maximum allowable outdoor standards.

One indoor air pollution study not only identified indoor air pollutants but verified that what you breathe travels throughout your body. Samples showed residues of gasoline on the breath of some people hours after they had filled their gas tanks, while a short visit to the dry cleaner resulted in tetrachloroethylene on the breath. Even taking a hot shower elevated breath levels of chloroform, which is released in the stream of chlorinated water. I can vouch for this. Earlier this afternoon, I ventured into the cleaning products aisle of a supermarket to check the warning label on a package of air freshener. In the time it took me to find the air freshener on the shelf—about two minutes—I could already taste in my mouth the toxic chemicals I was breathing that had escaped the sealed bottles of cleaning products.

HOW TO BE TOXIC-FREE

If your home has indoor air pollution, you may or may not need an air filter.

The preferred method of reducing indoor air pollution is to simply remove toxic air pollutants at their source. You will find many suggestions for doing just this throughout this book. Any recommendation with a nose icon will reduce indoor air pollutants that you inhale into your body.

And then increase ventilation. Keep your windows open as much as the weather allows and, even better, invest in a window fan. If you need more ventilation but don't want to lose heat or cool air, consider an air exchanger. For more information, contact a local heating, ventilation, and air-conditioning (HVAC) contractor: Look in the Yellow Pages of your telephone book under "Heating, Ventilation, and Air-conditioning."

If you can't solve your indoor air pollution problem by removing pollutants at their source or diluting them with added ventilation, then it's time to get an air filter.

Air filters can be purchased as portable models or you can have them built into your central heating/air-conditioning system. Keep in mind that the cleaning capacity of any portable unit is limited to the one room it is in.

To effectively filter your air, you need to buy the correct type of filter for the type of pollutants you need to remove. If you need to remove particles, your best choice is a HEPA filter. To remove gases, you want a carbon filter. Some filters contain both for broad spectrum removal of pollutants.

Truly effective portable air filters are rarely sold in stores, but are easily available on the Internet. For built-in whole-house filtration, check the Yellow Pages of your telephone book for an HVAC dealer.

Carbon Monoxide

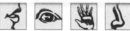

Warning: Natural gas, like many petroleum-based substances such as gasoline, naturally contains benzene, a chemical known to cause cancer. The benzene in natural gas is destroyed when gas is burned in appliances. A warning odorant is added to natural gas so that leaks of unburned gas can quickly be detected. If gas is detected, contact your local utility company promptly.

Warning: Soot and formaldehyde, which may be produced when natural gas is burned, are also chemicals known to cause cancer. Properly operating appliances reduces the formation of soot.

CARBON MONOXIDE is a by-product of burning natural gas, kerosene, or wood for cooking or to produce heat.

According to the U.S. Consumer Product Safety Commission, hundreds of people die from carbon monoxide poisoning each year in this country. Thousands of others suffer dizziness, nausea, and convulsions. You can't see, taste, or smell carbon monoxide. But it kills.

Carbon monoxide starves the body and brain of oxygen. First symptoms include sleepiness, headache, dizziness, flushed skin, disorientation, abnormal reflexes, blurred vision, irritability, and an inability to concentrate. As poisoning progresses, the victim experiences nausea and vomiting, shortness of breath, convulsions, unconsciousness, and finally death.

Many years ago, my grandmother almost died of carbon monoxide exposure from her faulty furnace.

Most cases of carbon monoxide poisoning at home involve gas appliances, such as kitchen ranges, space heaters, wall heaters, central heating systems, and clothes dryers.

HOW TO BE TOXIC-FREE

The key to catching carbon monoxide before it kills is early detection. But you don't need to wait until you or a loved one has symptoms.

Every home that has gas heat or any other gas appliance should have a carbon monoxide detector. They can be purchased at any hardware or home improvement store or on the Internet. Prices start at less than $20 online—a small price to pay for peace of mind.

Another option is to go all-electric. Electric ranges, heaters, water heaters, and clothes dryers do not emit carbon monoxide.

An affordable way to transition away from gas heat is to get some electric space heaters. These can be purchased at most hardware and home improvement stores during the winter season.

Look for heaters made with metal housings, not plastic, as plastic can emit toxic fumes when heated.

Here are some types of heaters with metal housings:

- ceramic "utility" heaters
- oil-filled "radiator" heaters
- "radiant" heaters with stainless steel housings

Plastics

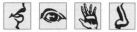

We use plastics in virtually every area of our lives. Plastics are a large, extremely diverse group of moldable synthetic materials made from petroleum or coal. They can be found as hard or soft solid forms, liquids that dry to solid coatings and finishes, adhesives, rigid or flexible foams, sheets, films, fibers, and filaments.

We are exposed to plastics in many different ways. There may be plastic vapors in the air we breathe; the plastic in clothing may rub against our skin; plastic from packaging and storage containers may be absorbed by our food; and plastic may be in the water we drink from plastic pipes or storage bottles.

There are many, many, many, many plastics. Each is different in its toxicity. When we say *plastic*, we are referring to a huge field of materials. So it's not really fair to say, "It's plastic, therefore it must be toxic," because that's just not a true statement. There are plastics that are very toxic, plastics that are pretty safe, and plastics that are in between.

Some types of plastics cause cancer, others are endocrine disruptors, and still others can cause skin rashes—perhaps a minor complaint, but still a sign from our bodies that something is wrong.

HOW TO BE TOXIC-FREE

Here are some easy guidelines to remember about plastics.

- **The form of the plastic makes a difference.** A single type of plastic can be used to make many different products. Various plasticizers are added to the basic formula to make the plastic softer. The general rule is that the harder the plastic, the less it outgases, and the softer the plastic, the more it outgases.
- **Heat causes plasticizers to outgas.** Whenever you expose a plastic to heat, it will release molecules of plasticizer. Conversely, cold

lessens the release of plasticizers. So if you have a case of plastic water bottles sitting in the sun on a truck or in front of a store, they are going to warm up and leach plastic into the water. Likewise, you don't want to use plastics anywhere where they will be heated.

- **Check the recycling symbol on the bottom of food containers.** Just remember: 1 PETE, 2 HDPE, 4 LDPE, and 5 PP are the safest. Forget the rest.

Don't worry about replacing *every* plastic product in your home: it's a virtually impossible task. My television, VCR, and telephone are all made largely from plastic, although my computer is made from aluminum and glass.

For the most part, however, you can live without plastic. Plastics have been popular only since World War II. Before that, everything was made from natural materials. There are many, many items still made from natural materials: wool diaper covers, wooden toys, straw baskets, cotton shower curtains, glass jars, and paper bags, to name just a few. So keep your eyes open, and when you have a choice, look for a natural material.

Household Cleaning and Laundry Products
Cleaning Products

Cleaning products are among the most toxic products you will find in your home—so much so that they are the only household products regulated by the Consumer Product Safety Commission under the 1960 Federal Hazardous Substances Labeling Act. This means that cleaning products that can hurt you must carry warnings on their labels.

If a cleaning product contains a chemical that is hazardous, by law it must prominently display the degree of toxicity with one of the following signal words:

- *Danger* (or *Poison*, with skull and crossbones): Could kill an adult if only a tiny pinch is ingested.
- *Warning:* Could kill an adult if about a teaspoon is ingested.
- *Caution:* Will not kill until an amount from 2 tablespoons to 2 cups is ingested.

At one time these signal words accurately indicated the dose required to cause a toxic effect, but because of poor labeling practices, these words now suggest only a general degree of danger.

The real safety or danger of cleaning products is difficult to assess because manufacturers are not required by law to list exact ingredients on the label. Most toxic ingredients in cleaning products are listed on the product's material safety data sheet (MSDS), but some are protected by trade secrets and even the government and poison control centers can't find out what they are.

HOW TO BE TOXIC-FREE

One of the easiest first steps you can take to being toxic-free is to replace all the toxic cleaners you have in your kitchen with toxic-free cleaning products. Just take a trip to the cleaning products section of your local natural-food store and you will find everything you need.

But you can also easily make your own cleaners from simple, inexpensive, and natural materials you probably already have in your kitchen. These replacements work every bit as well as the chemicals you are accustomed to using. They also have the added benefit of being much less expensive than commercial cleaning preparations. You don't have to pay for advertising or packaging or buy a different product for each cleaning need.

I do all my cleaning with a squirt bottle of equal parts vinegar and water plus organic liquid soap and baking soda.

I also have a steam cleaner. When plain water is turned into steam, it can literally melt away dirt, grease, grime, soap scum, mold, mildew, and calcium and lime deposits. You can clean, sanitize, and deodorize almost anything without scrubbing or chemicals.

You really can clean everything with simple formulas you make at home, and there are several good books with all the instructions. The easiest one to start with is *Clean House, Clean Planet: Clean Your House for Pennies a Day the Safe, Nontoxic Way* by Karen Logan.

Drain Cleaners

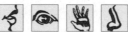

Poison: Call poison center, emergency room, or physician at once. Causes severe eye and skin damage; may cause blindness. Harmful or fatal if swallowed.

THE PRIMARY component of drain cleaners is **lye**, an extremely corrosive material that can eat right through skin. Even a drop spilled on your skin or a dry crystal that falls on wet skin can cause damage. When ingested, lye quickly burns through internal tissues, damaging the esophagus, the stomach, and the entire intestinal tract. The internal damage may be irreparable for those who survive lye poisoning.

Lye itself poses no danger from inhalation, but in liquid drain cleaners, lye is mixed with such volatile liquid chemicals as **ammonia** and **petroleum distillates**, which can release harmful vapors.

If you change only one cleaning product in your home, this is it. Drain cleaners get my vote for the most dangerous unnecessary product in the house.

HOW TO BE TOXIC-FREE

For all their dangers, lye-based drain cleaners are really not very effective. How many times have you tried to clear a drain with lye, only to have the clog just sit there, leaving you with a sink full of corrosive, lye-contaminated water and wondering what to do next? Why endanger your family with a product that doesn't even work?

My favorite drain opener is the handy-dandy plunger. This old-fashioned standby works nearly every time. You can buy one that will last for years at any hardware store, and they are very inexpensive. True, at times it takes more than a few plunges, but usually the clog will break down eventually.

If this doesn't work, lye won't work, either, so call a plumber. He will use a long, flexible metal snake to push the clog away. If the clog is farther down the pipe, use a device that creates water pressure with water from your garden hose to push the clog through. Look for them at your hardware or plumbing store.

The best solution, however, is preventive maintenance. Use a drain strainer to trap food particles and hair (I use the kind that are a fine mesh screen), and remember not to pour grease down the drain (dump it in the garbage or into a "grease can" instead). I really can't remember the last time we had a clogged drain.

OVEN CLEANERS

  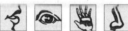

DANGER: Contact will cause burns. Avoid contact with skin, eyes, mucous membranes, and clothing. Do not take internally. Wear rubber gloves while using. Contains lye. If taken internally, or sprayed in eyes, call a physician. Keep out of reach of children. Irritant to mucous membranes. Avoid inhaling vapors.

ALTHOUGH OVEN cleaners contain several toxic ingredients, the greatest dangers come from **lye** and **ammonia**. Oven cleaners in **aerosol spray** containers are especially hazardous, because the spray sends tiny droplets of lye and ammonia into the air, where they can easily be inhaled or land in your eyes or on your skin.

Be especially wary of oven cleaners that advertise "no fumes." I have tried several brands, and all still smelled very strongly of ammonia.

HOW TO BE TOXIC-FREE

If you are like me, you probably don't like to clean your oven. It is possible to never have to clean your oven if you are very careful about not allowing things to spill. If your casserole seems like it might spill over during baking, put a cookie sheet or sheet of aluminum foil on the lower rack. On those rare occasions when something does end up on the bottom of the oven instead of on your plate, wipe it up as soon as the oven has cooled, to prevent it from baking on even more.

Still, accidents do happen. I know of no commercial toxic-free oven cleaners, but I'll give you a tip from a friend of mine who runs her own nontoxic cleaning service and refuses to use toxic chemicals. Here's how Gina cleans ovens.

GINA'S OVEN CLEANER

Mix together in a spray bottle 2 tablespoons liquid soap (not detergent), 2 teaspoons borax, and warm water to fill the bottle. Make sure the salts are completely dissolved to avoid clogging the squirting mechanism. Spray it on, holding the bottle very close to the oven surface so the solution doesn't get into the air (and into your eyes and lungs). Even though these are natural ingredients, this solution is designed to cut heavy-duty grime, so wear gloves and glasses or goggles, if you have them. Leave the solution on for 20 minutes, then scrub with steel wool and a nonchlorine scouring powder. Rub impossible, baked-on black spots with pumices, available in a stick at hardware stores.

IF YOU have an extremely dirty oven layered with years of baked-on grease, you may have to use a chemical oven cleaner *once* to get it clean before you can begin your nontoxic maintenance. For this *one* application, choose a nonaerosol product and follow these precautions from the Consumer Product Safety Commission for safer use of oven cleaners:

- Read the directions before each use and follow them.
- Wear protective gloves and goggles.
- Open windows in the kitchen and be sure that children and other members of the family are out of the room.
- If the fumes begin to affect you, close the oven door, leave the room, and get fresh air.

Mold and Mildew Cleaners

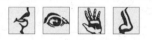

DANGER: Eye irritant. Keep out of reach of children. Use only in well-ventilated area.

MOLD AND mildew cleaners may contain **phenol**, **kerosene**, or **pentachlorophenol**, all of which may be harmful through skin absorption or inhalation, or fatal if swallowed. Labels warn that mold-and-mildew cleaners are a dangerous eye irritant, yet they are usually packed in either pump or aerosol spray containers, which send the harmful mist into the air.

HOW TO BE TOXIC-FREE

You can make your own mold-and-mildew cleaner by mixing borax and water, or vinegar and water, in a spray bottle. Spray it on and the mold wipes right off. Borax inhibits mold growth, so you can sprinkle it in damp areas, such as under the sink.

Mold is a common indoor air pollutant. Mold will only grow in a damp, dark environment, so it becomes a problem only in areas where it can proliferate because of excessive moisture. In most homes, this is the kitchen and the bathroom.

The best solution is to prevent mold growth in the first place by creating an environment that is dry and light. Look around your home for sources of moisture and fix them: no moisture, no mold. Controlling mold in a bathroom may involve running the exhaust fan after a shower to pull moisture out of the room. I installed a large skylight over my shower, which not only lets in light but keeps the bathroom dry.

Disinfectants

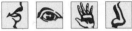

CAUTION: Keep out of reach of children. Keep away from heat, sparks, and open flame. Keep out of eyes. Avoid contact with food.

DISINFECTANTS CONTAIN a number of volatile chemicals that are dangerous to inhale. The ingredient most frequently found in disinfectants is **cresol**, a chemical easily absorbed through the skin and through the mucous membranes of the respiratory tract. Cresol can damage your liver, kidneys, lungs, pancreas, and spleen, and it is also a potent neurotoxicant. Disinfectants also may contain other toxic germ killers, such as **phenol**, **ethanol**, **formaldehyde**, **ammonia**, and **chlorine**.

Ironically, most people use a disinfectant when there is an illness in the family, just when the sick person is most vulnerable to toxic effects. Some people are so concerned about cleanliness that they overdisinfect and are constantly surrounded by that "fresh, clean smell"—actually dangerous fumes.

Nature, in her wondrous way, has provided our bodies with an effective immune system (see page 191) to process any germs that come our way. Use of toxic chemicals to kill germs can compromise the ability of the very system that exists to come to our defense.

HOW TO BE TOXIC-FREE

I personally use no disinfectants of any kind whatsoever, and haven't for over twenty years. Instead, I support my immune system with nutrition and rarely even catch a cold.

Disinfectants will, as the television commercials say, "kill germs on contact," but they will not kill *all* germs present, only some of them.

Germs are very friendly with one another and will quickly multiply soon after disinfecting.

If you want to eliminate disease-causing bacteria and viruses, you must sterilize items by immersing them in boiling water. This is how in hospitals surgical instruments are sterilized, with steam pressure in an autoclave.

One study I read about years ago showed that a solution of ½ cup borax dissolved in 1 gallon of hot water satisfied all the germicidal requirements of the hospital in which the study was conducted (I wish someone would replicate this study, as the original seems to be no longer available). Borax, which is available in the cleaning products department of your supermarket, is also recommended to add to diaper pails.

Regular cleaning with soap and water is also an effective way to reduce bacteria. Soap works by reducing the surface tension of water and allowing scrubbing action to loosen and carry away bacteria. Since friction is the key, the more you scrub—whether your skin or a countertop—the cleaner it will be. When surgeons scrub to sanitize their hands before surgery, they don't just rub on a little antibacterial soap, they *scrub* and *scrub* and *scrub* (for two minutes). A nurse I know told me that even ordinary hand washing should include a soapy twenty second scrub, about the time it takes to sing the little "ABC" song. And by the way, antibacterial soaps that contain toxic **triclosan** are not needed. Just a good, plain, unscented soap will do.

In the kitchen, we do need to be cognizant of some specific harmful microorganisms, such as salmonella in raw meats. I handle this without toxic chemicals by having a separate cutting board that I use only for meat, which then immediately gets washed in the hottest water, along with the knife I used and my hands. This is the method used in restaurants, which are inspected by the local health department. Restaurant supply houses sell color-coded boards to be used for different foods.

Even a rinse of hot water will kill some bacteria. And keep things dry—bacteria, mildew, and mold cannot live without dampness.

Spot Removers

CAUTION: Eye irritant. Vapor harmful. Keep out of reach of children.

THE MOST commonly used solvent in spot removers is **perchloroethylene**, the same solvent used in dry cleaning. Your major risk from perchloroethylene comes from exposure when actually using the product. Perchloroethylene fumes are carcinogenic, highly toxic, and can cause light-headedness, dizziness, sleepiness, nausea, loss of appetite, and disorientation. Exposure to large amounts of perchloroethylene fumes can be fatal.

HOW TO BE TOXIC-FREE

Spots are easiest to remove the minute they occur, so get in the habit of attacking spots when they happen, before they become stains.

Many years ago, my literary agent invited me to join her for dessert at a luncheon she was having in a fancy restaurant with an important editor from a major publishing house. I ordered an ice cream creation that was swimming in a pool of bittersweet chocolate sauce. I took one bite and the entire scoop of ice cream landed on the skirt of my red cotton corduroy dress. My agent immediately ordered a bottle of club soda and doused my dress thoroughly. It didn't all come out, but when I washed my dress later in plain soap and water, the chocolate stain entirely disappeared.

There are many less toxic commercial spot removers now available, sold at major retailers. Also check the Internet for do-it-yourself spot removal instructions.

Dry Cleaning

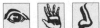

Many garments made from both natural and synthetic fibers are labeled "Dry clean only."

Dry cleaning isn't really "dry"; instead of detergent and water, items are "washed" with a solvent that removes spots and stains without being absorbed by the fiber. Dry-cleaned fabrics don't shrink or stretch, dyes don't fade or run, delicate fabrics don't tear or water-spot, and wools don't mat.

Dry-cleaned clothes carry no warning labels, but they should. Unless otherwise specified, the solvent is probably **perchloroethylene** (called "perc" in the industry). It is the most common solvent used in dry cleaning and the most toxic. It is considered to be a Group 2A carcinogen, which means that it is probably carcinogenic to humans. It is also a neurotoxicant and can cause liver damage. Perc is very volatile and can easily permeate anything porous, such as stuffed furniture and food. So clothing dry-cleaned with perchloroethylene is not a good thing to have around the house.

The second most common type of solvent used in dry cleaning is **hydrocarbon**. It is sometimes marketed as "organic" but that does NOT mean it is organically grown. *Organic* in this case refers to the type of chemical it is, namely, a chemical made from chains of carbon molecules. This is pure petroleum. Hydrocarbon solvents are classified as volatile organic chemicals (VOCs). They can vaporize into the atmosphere and contribute to smog and global warming. There are many types of hydrocarbon solvents. They are usually very toxic.

Other toxic chemicals that also may be used in the dry-cleaning process are **benzene, chlorine, formaldehyde, naphthalene, trichloroethylene**, and **xylene**.

HOW TO BE TOXIC-FREE

Do dry-cleaned items pose a hazard? Yes and no. Inhaling perchloroethylene fumes is dangerous, but perchloroethylene is a very volatile substance that evaporates thoroughly, leaving no residue. Dry-cleaned items do go through a drying process, but many times the items are still damp when covered with their protective plastic. Studies done by the EPA listed fumes from slightly damp dry-cleaned items as a common indoor air pollutant.

The solution is simple. As soon as you bring home dry-cleaned items, remove the plastic covering and hang them in a well-ventilated area (preferably outdoors) to encourage evaporation of the solvent. Close the door to keep fumes out of the rest of the house, and then open windows in the extra room to ventilate the solvent fumes to the outside.

But perc is toxic, and there are less toxic alternatives.

Some cleaners now also do "wet cleaning," which combines hand washing, spot cleaning, steaming, and high-tech washing machines (using only special detergents and water) and clothes dryers. The advantage to having your clothes washed at a dry cleaner instead of washing them at home is that computer-controlled dryers and stretching machines ensure that the fabric retains its natural size and shape.

There are also less toxic solvents being used for dry cleaning.

Glycol ethers are less toxic than other petroleum solvents but are still made from petroleum and still toxic.

Liquid silicone is essentially liquefied sand. It is made from one of the earth's safest and most abundant natural minerals, silica. In the environment, it simply returns to its three natural elements: sand and trace amounts of water and CO_2. It is so safe it is not even regulated.

Liquid CO_2 is the safest choice for dry cleaning. CO_2 is the gas that all animals exhale and plants breathe in a high-pressure liquid form. It's the same stuff used to carbonate soda. It is used along with detergent. It cleans and disinfects garments. It flushes through fabrics to rid them of dirt particles and prevent stains from setting, and even flushes out harmful chemicals left behind by other dry cleaners. CO_2 cleaning can extend the life of the clothing from 20 percent to 40 percent.

The CO_2 used for dry cleaning is captured as a by-product of existing industrial processes, utilizing emissions that would otherwise be released into the atmosphere. Only about 2 percent of the CO_2 is lost into the air with each load of clothing, so it's impact on global warming is minimal. CO_2 dry cleaning is recognized by the EPA and Natural Resources Defense Council (NRDC) as a truly green dry-cleaning method, and rated number one by *Consumer Reports* for effectiveness—even better than conventional dry cleaning. There are not a lot of CO_2 dry cleaners, but those that exist are listed at www.findco2.com.

When evaluating a dry cleaner that claims to be less toxic, it's important to ask what solvents are used. CO_2 can be used with a nontoxic detergent or glycol ethers, for example. So check out cleaners thoroughly, and don't just rely on their advertising claims.

Of course, you can always wash any garment by hand instead of taking it to the dry cleaner, and also choose clothing that doesn't need to be dry-cleaned. I buy only clothing I can toss in the washer or wash by hand.

But I also understand that some clothing does need to be professionally cleaned, like business suits. In that case, choose the least toxic option available to you.

Laundry: Detergents, Bleach, and Fabric Softeners

DETERGENT WARNING

Danger: In case of eye contact, get prompt medical attention. Keep out of reach of children.

Warning: Harmful if swallowed, irritating to eyes and skin. Keep out of reach of children.

BLEACH WARNING

Caution: Keep out of reach of children. May be harmful if swallowed or may cause severe eye irritation. Never mix chlorine bleach with cleaning products containing ammonia, or with vinegar. The resulting chloramine fumes are deadly.

FABRICS SOFTENER WARNING

Caution: Keep out of reach of children.

PLEASE NOTE that all three common laundry product labels say "Keep out of reach of children." Yet, most parents leave these products sitting out where children *can* reach them. As a result, detergents are responsible for more household poisonings than any other household product, most often when children accidentally ingest colorful powders packaged in easy-to-open boxes.

Detergents also leave residues on clothing and bedsheets, which can cause severe rashes, and artificial "springtime-fresh" fragrances can cause a multitude of symptoms.

Chlorine bleach is hazardous both by accidental ingestion and from fumes inhaled during use. Product labels warn only against drinking liquid bleach, but toxicology books report that chlorine is "toxic as a skin irritant and by inhalation."

Fabric softeners leave a residue on fabrics to control static cling. They never really wash out, so you are constantly exposed whenever you are in contact with a fabric. Residues can be very irritating to skin and cause allergic reactions such as stuffy nose and watery eyes. Fabric softeners also are usually very strongly scented and contain many ingredients that are neurotoxic.

HOW TO BE TOXIC-FREE

Detergent

There is a big difference between detergent and soap.

Detergents are formulated from petroleum. Soap, on the other hand, is made from natural oils and minerals and has been safely used for centuries.

Natural and organic soap-based laundry products can be found in natural-food stores and online.

There's also a new laundry product called soapnuts. These are actual unprocessed nuts that, when placed in water, create a soaplike substance that cleans and softens fabrics. They really work. I use them myself.

The new high-efficiency front-loading washing machines require low-sudsing detergents. Regular detergents, even in reduced amounts, still produce too many suds. Most of the plant-based laundry products sold in natural-food stores can be used in front-loading washers. In fact, a common complaint about plant-based laundry products in general is that they *don't* suds as much as we are accustomed to with supermarket detergents. Check the labels on brands sold in your local natural-food store.

You may not even need to use any laundry product to get your clothes clean. Often the purpose of laundering is not so much to get rid of dirt as to freshen clothing and remove perspiration and odors. For this you can use about a cup of baking soda or white vinegar per washload.

Bleach

Clothes start to look dull and dingy because the minerals in hard water make soap and detergent stick to fabrics, producing a film that dulls colors and turns whites gray. Simply using a water softener can solve the problem. No bleach is needed. Baking soda works fine. Just add enough so the water feels "slippery."

I have a whole-house salt-free water conditioner because I live in an area that has very hard water, so I don't need to use bleach. But if you do, choose a nonchlorine, unscented "oxygen" bleach product made from hydrogen peroxide and sodium carbonate. These are available everywhere laundry products are sold. They often have the prefix *oxy-* in the name or are referred to as "nonchlorine" bleaches. Read the labels carefully, though. Some "nonchlorine" bleaches contain artificial fragrance.

Oxygen bleaches are also good for other uses. I've used it to remove old stains from clothing that I hadn't been able to get out using other methods. It also removed stains and pot marks from my sink and the tea stain from the bottom of my favorite teacup. It makes my toilet and tile sparkle. In short, it's a great toxic-free substitute for anything you would want to clean with chlorine bleach.

Fabric Softener

Fabric softeners didn't even exist before synthetic fibers became popular. They were developed solely to reduce the static cling that builds up on synthetic fabrics. If you wear natural fibers, you don't need to use fabric softener at all, because there is no problem with static cling. If you do need a fabric softener, the safest and most convenient type is the unscented sheet variety that goes into the dryer. Baking soda added to the rinse cycle also acts as a fabric softener.

Glass Cleaners

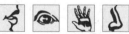

Poison: May cause burns. Call a physician. Keep out of reach of children.

Caution: Harmful if swallowed. Irritant. Avoid contact with eyes and prolonged contact with skin. Do not swallow. Avoid inhalation of vapors. Use in a well-ventilated area.

MANY PEOPLE assume that **ammonia** is safe because our grandmothers used it, but it's not. The warning labels above are found on bottles of full-strength ammonia. It's a toxic substance.

Window cleaners contain ammonia mixed with water and artificial coloring.

And because they come in a spray bottle, these tiny droplets of diluted ammonia can end up on your skin and in your eyes and lungs.

HOW TO BE TOXIC-FREE

An easy way to begin to eliminate ammonia from your home is to wash your windows with distilled white or apple cider vinegar, mixed in equal parts with water in a spray bottle. Squirt on windows and wipe with recycled newspapers for a streak-free super shine.

If you have a bottle of ammonia under your sink for other cleaning purposes, take it to a household hazardous waste collection site. Yes, your local garbage company doesn't want you to put it in the garbage. It's that toxic.

Then go to your local natural-food store and pick up an ammonia-free all-purpose cleaner made from natural plant-based ingredients.

Air Fresheners

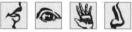

KEEP OUT OF REACH OF CHILDREN
Caution: Eye and skin irritant. Prolonged or frequent skin contact may cause allergic reaction. Avoid contact with eyes, skin, and clothing. Do not ingest.

A FRIEND and I were out shopping when I said I needed to stop and look for the warning label on air fresheners. "They shouldn't call these air fresheners," he said. "They should be called air toxifiers." And that's exactly correct, for air fresheners do add toxic chemicals to the air.

Most air fresheners don't "freshen" the air at all: They cover up the offensive odor with a more pleasant one, or interfere with your ability to smell by releasing a nerve-deadening agent or coating your nasal passages with an undetectable film.

In 2007 the Natural Resources Defense Council did a study on air fresheners and found that more than 85 percent of the samples tested contained various amounts of **phthalates**. This group of chemicals is used to dissolve and carry fragrances, soften plastics, among other things, and are commonly found in a variety of products, including cosmetics, paints, nail polish, and children's toys.

Health effects connected with phthalates are cancer, developmental and sex-hormone abnormalities (including decreased testosterone and sperm levels and malformed sex organs) in infants, and infertility. Currently there are no regulations on phthalates, and the labeling of phthalate content on products is not required.

Other toxicants frequently found in air fresheners are **naphthalene**, **phenol**, **cresol**, **ethanol**, **xylene**, and **formaldehyde**.

HOW TO BE TOXIC-FREE

Air freshener is one of those products that is highly advertised but probably completely unnecessary.

You can rid your home of undesirable odors simply by opening a window or turning on an exhaust fan such as the one in the hood over your stove. This will also help reduce any toxic fumes that are building up indoors.

Track down odors in your home, find out what's causing them, and handle the odor at the source. To reduce food smells, empty the garbage frequently and clean the can when needed.

If you have heavy-duty odors to remove, try zeolite. Zeolites are a complex group of naturally occurring minerals, most of which are derived from volcanic ash. They have a complex lattice structure which is arranged in a honeycomb-like framework. The channels provide enormous internal surface areas within the zeolite crystals, which are lined with negatively charged ions and have a natural electrostatic attraction to positively charged pollutants. Zeolites are widely used industrially for odor control and to remove toxic substances from the air. You can order zeolite online.

If your main reason for using an air freshener is to scent the air, try natural fragrances instead. Use the real thing if you can (right at the moment I'm enjoying the lovely scent of real paperwhite narcissus sitting on my desk), or make your own air freshener spray by adding essential oil to water in a spray bottle. Also look for air fresheners made with natural essential oils.

There are also products designed to eliminate odors on "soft" household surfaces—such as mattresses and box springs, carpets and rugs, curtains and drapes, pet areas, and upholstered furniture—that can be difficult to clean and deodorize. These are made from ethyl alcohol (distilled from petrochemicals) with added fragrance. However, you can do the same thing all-natural, without the scent, for much less money, by simply putting straight vodka in an atomizer.

Household Pest Control
Household Insecticides

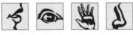

Caution: Keep out of reach of children. Use only when area to be treated is vacated by humans and pets. Not to be taken internally by humans or animals. Hazardous if swallowed or absorbed through skin. Do not get on skin, in eyes, or on clothing. Avoid breathing of vapors or spray mist. Do not smoke while using. Should not be used in homes of the seriously ill or those on medication. Should not be used in homes of pollen-sensitive people or asthmatics. Do not use in any rooms where infants, the sick, or aged are or will be present for any extended period of confinement. Do not use in kitchen areas or areas where food is prepared or served. Do not apply directly to food. In the home, all food-processing surfaces and utensils should be covered during treatment or thoroughly washed before use. Remove pets, and cover fish aquariums and delicate plants before spraying.

ACCORDING TO the EPA, no insecticides that are sold for general home use have warning labels stronger than "Caution." Any products that pose greater danger are available only for application by licensed pest-control operators.

Most insecticides kill all types of flying and crawling insects: ants, fleas, cockroaches, mosquitoes, flies, and silverfish.

HOW TO BE TOXIC-FREE

Even though I live in Florida, a subtropical paradise where there are lots of bugs, I rarely have problems with insects inside my house that require even natural pest-control methods. Why? I keep my house well protected by using screens on windows and doors, and closing up any cracks and openings where pests could enter.

Here's how I eliminated the ant problem in my house. When you see a trail of ants, wipe them up with a wet sponge. Ants rely on one another for direction. Without a trail, others get lost. See where they are coming into your house, and seal up that crack with ordinary white glue (it will dry clear and invisible). You may need to do this a few times as ants come into your house, but eventually all your cracks will be sealed and no more ant problem.

I highly recommend that you find toxic-free alternatives for any household insecticide you are using. My favorite book on the subject is *Tiny Game Hunting: Environmentally Healthy Ways to Trap and Kill the Pests in Your House and Garden* by Hilary Dole Klein and Adrian M. Wenner.

The Pesticide Action Network (www.pesticideinfo.org) maintains an extensive database of pesticides, pesticide products, least toxic alternatives, and additional resources.

Insect Repellents

Caution: Harmful if swallowed. Avoid contact with eyes and lips. Do not allow children to rub eyes if hands have been treated. Do not apply on or near: rayon, spandex, or other synthetics. May damage furniture finishes, plastics, leather, watch crystals, and painted or varnished surfaces including automobiles.

I DON'T know about you, but I don't think I'd want to rub something on my skin that could take the paint off my car!

The most commonly used pesticide in insect repellents is **DEET** (common name for **N,N-diethyl-meta-toluamide**). According to the British medical journal *The Lancet*, exposure to DEET has been reported to cause brain disorders, slurred speech, difficulty walking, tremors, and even death. *Consumer Reports* has documented at least a dozen cases of acute neurotoxicity in children who had been exposed to or accidentally swallowed DEET. Some of the children died.

Obviously, while not everyone who uses a DEET-based insect repellent will suffer these effects, it makes you think twice, especially since up to 56 percent of DEET enters the bloodstream after it is applied to the surface of your skin, and it can remain in your body for up to two months.

HOW TO BE TOXIC-FREE

Most people use insect repellents to keep mosquitoes away. We have a lot of mosquitoes here in Florida, so keeping mosquitoes off my body is something I know about.

The easiest mosquito repellant is plain vinegar. I use organic apple cider vinegar because that's what I have in my kitchen, but you could also use distilled white vinegar. I just put it in an oil-and-vinegar shaker-type bottle, which I can use to shake the vinegar drop by drop onto exposed areas.

I've also had success with various herbal insect repellants and cedar oil, which you can order on the Internet.

I've also used cotton mosquito netting, also available on the Internet.

Mothballs

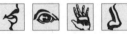

Caution: May be harmful if swallowed. Avoid prolonged breathing of vapor or repeated contact with skin. Keep out of reach of children.

MOTHBALLS ARE made from 100 percent **paradichlorobenzene**, a volatile toxic chemical that can cause headaches and severe irritation to nose, throat, and lungs. Over time, it can cause liver and kidney damage.

Because the balls look like candy, they are a very attractive poison to children. If a two-year-old were to eat even one mothball accidentally, he or she could develop seizures in less than an hour.

It has always seemed inconsistent to me that the warning label on mothballs says "Avoid prolonged breathing of vapor," yet mothballs by their very design give off these fumes. The odor of mothballs hidden in a closet can easily permeate an entire bedroom and increase to very high levels if the room is not ventilated adequately.

HOW TO BE TOXIC-FREE

Protect your woolens from moths by making sachets from dried lavender, equal parts dried rosemary and mint, or whole peppercorns. Cedar products are also effective moth repellants.

Not only are these herbal products safe and effective, but their natural scent is far more pleasant.

Make sure the herbal products contain ingredients of natural origin, and not artificial fragrances.

Here's a tip to make an easy sachet: Use cotton baby socks! They are just the right size and many have pretty designs. Just fill the "foot" with herbs, fold the top over, and secure with a safety pin.

Lice Shampoo

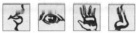

Every parent with a school-age child might someday have to deal with a child picking up head lice at school.

At one time the most common treatment for head lice was a shampoo that contained **lindane**, a very toxic chemical easily absorbed through the skin. One child's death was reported to have been the result of lindane poisoning after treatment for head lice, and lindane now is known to cause convulsions, seizures, and cancer in laboratory animals.

While shampoos containing lindane are still sold, the preferred active ingredient nowadays is pyrethrin, which is the crushed, dried flowers of *Chrysanthemum cinerariifolium*. It's harmless to humans and pets, but kills bugs on contact. The toxicity problem is not with pyrethrin itself but with the added **petroleum distillates**. Because the specific petroleum distillates are not identified (and usually not even known to the manufacturer, as "petroleum distillates" are sold as a mix of whatever chemicals of that type are available on any given day), I would hesitate to put chemicals of unknown toxicity on my child's scalp, especially since the scalp area is very porous, and chemicals put on the hair are easily absorbed into the bloodstream.

HOW TO BE TOXIC-FREE

The National Pediculosis Association (www.headlice.org) is dedicated to protecting children from the misuse and abuse of potentially harmful lice and scabies pesticidal treatments. Visit their website to find out about toxic-free standardized head lice management programs to keep the children in school lice- and nit-free.

Water
Shower Filters

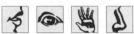

It's important to drink pure water, but as an inexpensive first step, it's actually more important to get a filter to remove toxic chemicals from the water in your shower.

Almost half of water pollutant exposure occurs *through the skin* in children and 50 to 70 percent in adults! Only about 20 to 50 percent of water pollutants ingested are actually taken into the body, but through the skin, virtually 100 percent of the contaminants go directly into the bloodstream.

So, filter your shower water, please.

The most common water pollutants are **chlorine** and **chloramines**, which must be added to water supplies as a disinfectant to protect public health from diseases caused by bacteria, viruses, and other organisms.

The major problem with chlorine is that when it combines with the natural organic matter in water (such as dead leaves), it forms **trihalomethanes (THMs)**, the most common of which is chloroform. Chloroform can cause liver and kidney damage and depress the nervous system, and it also causes cancer. According to the EPA, trihalomethanes have been present in virtually all chlorinated water supplies. And they have identified chloroform released from hot, running shower water as a major indoor *air pollutant*, so there is a hazard in breathing shower steam too.

For this reason and others, chlorine is now being replaced by chloramines. Chloramines come with a warning label not to use water treated with them in your fish tank, as it will kill the fish.

HOW TO BE TOXIC-FREE

The solution is to get a shower filter. Most shower filters contain activated carbon or a metallic powder called KDF. Both will remove chlorine. Find them on the Internet for less than $50.

If you need to remove chloramines from your shower water, you'll need a filter with carbon designed especially for that purpose.

Call your local water provider to find out if your water contains chlorine or chloramines before purchasing a shower filter.

Bottled Water and Water Bottles

Though all bottled waters are required to meet EPA standards for drinking water and be labeled with standard definitions, there is a big toxic-exposure problem with bottled water: the bottle itself.

Most clear plastic bottles in which spring and drinking water is sold contain **bisphenol A (BPA)**, a potent endocrine disruptor that can impair reproductive organs and hormones and have adverse effects on breast tissue and prostate glands.

While it's good for your health to carry your own water and drink it throughout the day, if that water is in a clear polycarbonate plastic bottle, it is leaching a toxic substance into your water—even if the bottle is sitting on a table at room temperature.

Is there a level of BPA that may be acceptable? We have to ask:

Acceptable to whom? A healthy male? A woman? A child? The elderly? And how would you know how much leaching has occurred in the water? It could easily vary from day to day, depending on how long the water had been in the bottle, and whether or not the sun was shining on the bottle in the delivery truck.

I'd rather be safe than sorry.

HOW TO BE TOXIC-FREE

The only bottled water I consider to be safe is water sold in glass bottles. The best idea, however, is to carry your own water that you place in a refillable bottle.

Because piles of plastic bottles are an environmental problem as well as a health risk, there are now many refillable water bottles for you to choose from.

I use glass bottles, as they do not leach anything harmful into the water. They are heavier to carry but are the safest choice. I fill them with water from my water filter.

BPA-free plastic and metal water bottles are widely available, but I have some concern that plastics and metals can leach into water from these as well.

I stick with glass as the safest and most hygienic material for water storage.

Beauty and Hygiene
Beauty and Hygiene Products

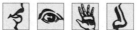

Beauty and hygiene products are used on some of the more sensitive parts of your body. You apply these products day in and day out, year after year, on your skin, which very easily absorbs whatever toxic ingredients these products contain; then they go right into your bloodstream and are rushed throughout your body in mere moments.

You would think these products would be tested for safety according to regulations as strict as those for the food we eat. Unfortunately, they are not.

Not surprisingly, the most common complaint associated with body-care products is skin rash, which can range in intensity from moderately irritating to painful and disfiguring. But beauty products also have other hazards. Did you know many lipsticks contain **lead**? Or that an accidental swallow from that bottle of perfume sitting on your dresser could kill your child?

Way back in 1989, at a government hearing on the safety of cosmetics, numerous cosmetologists testified about symptoms such as headaches, loss of balance, memory loss, asthma, and irreparable nervous system and respiratory problems as a result of working with cosmetics. Because of these testimonies, a House subcommittee asked the National Institute for Occupational Safety and Health (NIOSH) to analyze 2,983 chemicals used at that time in cosmetics. NIOSH found that 884 of the ingredients were found to be toxic.

Today it is easy to sort out which body-care products are toxic and which are not. Just visit Skin Deep, the Environmental Working Group's cosmetics safety database (www.cosmeticsdatabase.com). It lists thousands of brand-name beauty products and ingredients and rates their toxicity, so you can look up what you are using and choose less toxic products.

For more information on toxic chemicals and the cosmetic industry, read *Not Just a Pretty Face: The Ugly Side of the Beauty Industry* by Stacy Malkan, and visit her website the Campaign for Safe Cosmetics (www.safecosmetics.org).

HOW TO BE TOXIC-FREE

I am happy to report that there are more natural beauty and hygiene products than ever before, they are getting purer and purer, they are easier to find, and they are more aesthetically pleasing. Now many beauty and hygiene products are even made with organically grown ingredients.

Start by looking for natural and organic body-care products in your local natural-food store. Most have a good selection of everything from soap, shampoo, and toothpaste to complete makeup collections. These products can be reasonably relied upon to be made primarily from plant, animal, and mineral ingredients, though few are completely petrochemical-free and the plant ingredients are usually grown with pesticides. This is why you want to take that extra step and look for beauty products with organically grown ingredients.

Also, look around your local community for salons and spas that use organic products. They use and sell products that are for professional use only that I have found to be more effective than many of the standard over-the-counter consumer beauty products. The best shampoo I've ever used, made with organic ingredients, I get from my hairdresser. It costs $25 for the bottle, but it's so concentrated, it lasts four months and makes my hair look great. I also get facials from an aesthetician who uses only products with organic ingredients, which again seem expensive until I see how long they last and how beautiful my skin looks.

And many of the purest beauty products are made by hand by small suppliers. Many of these are sold on the Internet (see www.debraslist .com).

You can also make many beauty and hygiene products yourself at home. There are many books with recipes for making everything from facials to toothpaste. The Campaign for Safe Cosmetics has some recipes to get you started on their website. For more, just search online for "make your own cosmetics."

It's mostly a matter of getting back to the basics and using organic products. I have greatly reduced the number of beauty products I used to use. I now use only handmade soap on my body, organic cleanser and moisturizer on my face, organic shampoo on my hair, and a small collection of natural cosmetics that I use only when I dress for business or special occasions (I've found some men don't like to kiss lipstick or hug women if they are going to get makeup on their shirt, so I go natural and choose the hugs and kisses over the makeup). That's all.

All the top fashion magazines and the most beautiful women in the world agree that you are the most beautiful you can be when your body is healthy and fit and you use beauty products to enhance your own beauty, rather than drastically changing the way you look. *The Truth About Beauty: Transform Your Looks and Your Life from the Inside Out* by Kat James is a good introduction to what you can do to make your body more naturally beautiful.

And then, of course, there is always the inner glow that shines through that is the most beautiful of all.

Hair Spray

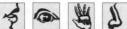

Warning: Flammable. Avoid fire, flame, or smoking during application and until hair is fully dry. Avoid spraying near eyes. Contents under pressure. Do not puncture or incinerate. Do not store at temperatures above 120 degrees F. Keep out of reach of children. Use only as directed. Intentional misuse by deliberately concentrating and inhaling contents can be harmful or fatal.

COMMON INGREDIENTS in hair spray include **aerosol propellants, alcohol, carcinogenic polyvinylpyrrolidone (PVP) plastic, formaldehyde**, and **artificial fragrance**.

Regular users of hair spray run the risk of developing a lung disease called thesaurosis, which causes enlarged lymph nodes, lung masses, and changes in blood cells. Fortunately, the disease is reversible. An FDA report noted that in one study, more than half of the women afflicted with this disease recovered within six months after discontinuing hair spray use.

Many people have allergic skin reactions to hair spray that ends up on delicate facial skin instead of on the hair. Eye and nasal irritations are also common side effects.

HOW TO BE TOXIC-FREE

I haven't used hair spray in more than twenty-five years (except on rare occasions when I'm on television and the makeup artist insists). For everyday, I just get a really good haircut that looks good without any styling aids.

I've noticed, too, that using a good organic shampoo that I get from my hairdresser makes a lot of difference in how my hair looks and handles. Though these shampoos cost more, I use so little that it actually costs less than buying multiple bottles of less expensive shampoo, and my hair looks and feels great.

If you do need to use hair spray, check your local natural-food store for an unscented natural hair spray in a nonaerosol pump spray bottle. These are much safer than the standard brands in the aerosol can but still may contain alcohol, artificial fragrance, and other ingredients that can cause allergic reactions in some people.

If you want to make your own hair spray at home, you can do so by putting 2 to 5 teaspoons of honey in a spray mist pump dispenser with about a cup of warm water and shake well. You'll have to experiment a bit with the proportions. The more honey it contains, the greater the holding power, but too much honey will make your hair sticky. Store the mixture in the refrigerator.

Mouthwash

Warning: Do not administer to children under 12 years of age. KEEP THIS AND ALL DRUGS OUT OF REACH OF CHILDREN. This product contains alcohol. Do not swallow. In case of accidental overdose, seek professional assistance or contact a poison control center immediately.

MOUTHWASH IS one of those everyday products that we assume to be safe, yet it is especially hazardous to children. Because we think it is safe, mouthwash is often left out where children can reach it, and it has an appealing color and taste. A child could easily drink enough to cause harm.

Mouthwash in general has a higher alcohol content than beer, wine, and many liquors! Beer is generally 4 to 10 percent, wine is 6 to 23 percent, depending on type, and mouthwash ranges from about 18 to 26 percent.

But here is something even worse: the alcohol in mouthwash is *denatured,* which means that other chemicals have been added to make it undrinkable (this is only because drinkable alcohol is subject to federal excise tax). Clearly, mouthwash is not intended to be an alcoholic beverage, but if your child drinks it accidentally, his or her body will respond as if they had just swallowed a very stiff drink. If too much is taken, your child could go into shock or a coma, possibly resulting in death.

Mouthwash is one of those products that is easy to make assumptions about. You would think that if a product is intended for use in the mouth, it would also be safe to swallow. I was surprised to see the label warn against this. It just goes against common sense.

Many mouthwashes also contain the antibacterial agent **triclosan**, a suspected carcinogen and known endocrine disruptor.

HOW TO BE TOXIC-FREE

Mouthwash is advertised to prevent bad breath, but actually what it does is kill bacteria in your mouth. It's not considered to be a replacement for brushing and flossing, but an extra precaution.

I don't know that mouthwash is necessary. I myself have never used mouthwash, I don't have bad breath, and I have never had a cavity. I do brush and floss.

If you do feel that you need to use a mouthwash, look for a brand made with natural ingredients at your natural-food store or on the Internet. But do keep it out of reach of children.

Toothpaste

Warning: Keep out of reach of children under 6 years of age. If you accidentally swallow more toothpaste than used for brushing, seek professional help or contact a poison control center immediately.

ORDINARY TOOTHPASTES can contain toxic chemicals such as **formaldehyde**, **polyvinylpyrrolidone** (**PVP**, a plastic), and **artificial colors and**

flavors, but the most toxic chemical of all in toothpaste is **fluoride**. Check the label. There's a warning.

Fluoride toothpastes and mouthwashes are often given to children as added protection against tooth decay. While there is no question that the optimal dose of fluoride can help prevent cavities, there is a possible danger that with the combination of fluoride in mouthwash, toothpaste, and tap water, children might be getting *too much* fluoride, causing mottling of the teeth and common ills such as headaches, tiredness, wrinkled skin, hair loss, thyroid problems, cancer, and many other disorders. And adults don't need fluoride at all.

HOW TO BE TOXIC-FREE

Toss that toxic toothpaste and look for a toothpaste or tooth powder that contains natural ingredients. Most do not contain fluoride. If they do, a natural brand is likely to contain naturally occurring sodium fluoride rather than fluoride that is waste from industrial manufacturing.

You can also stop using toothpaste altogether and brush your teeth with baking soda, either plain or flavored with a few drops of your favorite extract or essential oil.

Brushing with plain water works fine too. The point is to get the food out from between your teeth so it doesn't cause tooth decay.

You might also want to look for a toothpaste that does not contain **sodium lauryl sulfate** (labeled "SLS-free"). Sodium lauryl sufate is a surfactant commonly used in toothpastes, soaps, shampoos, and other products that "foam up." SLS is highly irritating to the skin, but can also cause hormone imbalances and cancer. It can enter your body through your skin and be stored in your heart, liver, lungs, and brain.

There's a fairly new product known as "tooth soap." It's not a paste or gel but rather shreds of actual soap. Users swear by it. If you want to try tooth soap, buy tooth soap designed for this use, or choose a plain soap without perfumes or colors.

Nail Polish and Nail Polish Remover

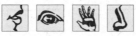

SINCE NAIL polish remover is the product that shows a warning label, let's start with that. The primary ingredient in most nail polish removers is the solvent **acetone**, which can not only dissolve nail polish but can cause your nails to become brittle and split, and skin rashes to develop on your fingers. When inhaled, the fumes from nail polish remover can irritate your lungs and make you feel light-headed. When accidentally ingested, acetone can cause restlessness and vomiting, and can result in a collapse into unconsciousness.

Nail polish is even more toxic but, amazingly, doesn't have a warning label. Nail polish contains **phenol**, **toluene**, and **xylene**, three highly volatile and harmful chemicals, but its basic ingredient is a **formaldehyde** resin.

HOW TO BE TOXIC-FREE

I personally don't wear nail polish, but I do like to have pretty nails. There's an inexpensive product called a nail buffer, which you can get at any drugstore, that gives your nails a satiny smooth surface and a glossy brilliant shine that last several days. I love the way my nails feel when I use the nail buffer—I like being able to make my nails look pretty without any toxic substances at all.

There now are also some "less toxic" nail polishes that do not have the most toxic solvents but are still made from plastics, and I just don't want to coat my nails with plastic. You can find them in many natural-food stores and on the Internet.

Perfume and Aftershave

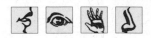

Perfumes and aftershave lotions are products that should be labeled "Keep out of reach of children" but aren't. According to my local poison control center, because of the high **alcohol** content of these products, it takes only about a tablespoon ingested accidentally for a small child to become intoxicated. This leads to lowered blood sugar, which can cause unconsciousness, and eventually the child could fall into a coma and die—all from one tablespoon of your favorite fragrance.

Perfume consists of a combination of natural essential oils, aroma, chemicals, and solvents in a base of alcohol. Some of these less-than-romantic ingredients include **methylene chloride, toluene, methyl ethyl ketone, methyl isobutyl ketone, ethanol**, and **benzyl chloride**—all designated as hazardous waste-disposal chemicals. In 1989, from a list of 2,983 chemicals used in the fragrance industry, the National Institute for Occupational Safety and Health (NIOSH) recognized 884 toxic substances capable of causing cancer, birth defects, central nervous system disorders, allergic reactions, skin and eye irritations, and chemical sensitivities.

"Fragrance" on a cosmetic label can indicate the presence of up to four thousand separate ingredients. Many of these chemicals are not listed on the label and protected under trade secrecy. Approximately 95 percent of these ingredients are derived from **petrochemicals**.

We have Coco Chanel to thank for perfume and fragrances made from synthetic petrochemical ingredients. Before Chanel No. 5 was introduced in 1921, all perfumes were made from natural ingredients. Chanel wanted a fragrance that was abstract, unique, and did not smell like any particular flower. Serendipitously, her chosen perfumer had been experimenting with synthetic fragrance molecules called aldehydes, which he mixed with a composition of essential flower oils to make a complex mixture of the natural and the man-made that is Chanel No. 5.

In 2010, the Campaign for Safe Cosmetics released a report called

Not So Sexy: The Health Risks of Secret Chemicals in Fragrance (www.safecos metics.org/downloads/NotSoSexy_report_May2010.pdf). They commissioned an independent lab to test seventeen fragrance products. They found four hormone-disrupting chemicals linked to a range of health effects, including sperm damage, thyroid disruption, and cancer. They noted that the majority of chemicals found have never been assessed for safety by any publically accountable agency or by the cosmetics industry's review panels.

When sprayed or applied on the skin, many chemicals in perfumes and other scented products are inhaled or absorbed through the skin. Perfume ingredients have even been found in the umbilical cord blood of newborn infants.

HOW TO BE TOXIC-FREE

I gave up perfume many years ago after I discovered I didn't have headaches if I didn't wear perfume or use scented products with synthetic fragrances.

If you want to wear a personal fragrance or use scented products, choose products made with natural essential oils.

Antiperspirants and Deodorants

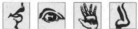

Antiperspirants may contain **aerosol propellants**, **ammonia**, **alcohol**, **formaldehyde**, and **fragrance**, but the primary danger is the active ingredient that helps stop wetness: **aluminum chlorohydrate**.

Aluminum chlorohydrate can cause infections in the hair follicles of your armpits, and skin irritations that can be severe enough to require medical attention. There is some concern as to whether the aluminum salts in antiperspirants contribute to a buildup of aluminum in the body (aluminum from other sources has been associated with various brain disorders) and about the safety of using aluminum in an aerosol spray. Because aerosols produce airborne particles that are likely to be inhaled, there is a good chance that bits of aluminum will enter the lungs and accumulate over time.

Non-antiperspirant deodorants may contain the bacteria-killing ingredient **triclosan**, which can cause liver damage when absorbed through the skin.

HOW TO BE TOXIC-FREE

There are a number of natural deodorants on the market, but what works best is baking soda—plain baking soda. I have recommended baking soda to a number of people who have suffered for many years with unconquerable body odor, and they say it's the only thing that has worked for them. Just take a bit of dry baking soda on your fingertips and pat it under your arms after you've dried off from your shower. Your skin should be slightly damp but not wet. If the baking soda feels too abrasive to you, you can mix it with cornstarch or white clay.

But you may not need a deodorant at all. It makes sense to me that the body in its natural state would smell good, as do other things in nature, and that a bad odor would be a symptom of something wrong with a body. One day I just stopped using baking soda as a deodorant— I had been using it because of advertising—and found I actually didn't need it. I didn't think my body smelled bad, and nobody cringes or pulls away when they get near me. Now I think body odor is a sign a body needs a detox (see Chapter 4), not a deodorant.

Body Soap

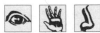

Soap has such a "clean" image, it's hard to imagine that it might contain some ingredients that are harmful to health.

Basically, all soap—whether intended for use on the body or for cleaning—is made from a combination of animal or vegetable fat and the mineral **sodium hydroxide (lye)**. Though sodium hydroxide is extremely hazardous—a single crystal can eat right through wet skin—don't worry: by the time the soap-making process is complete, all the molecules have broken down and recombined into a smooth, safe cleanser. Natural glycerin, a by-product of this combination, is also used as a base for soap. Herbs, scents, colors, and other ingredients can be added to either type of soap.

Because the Food and Drug Administration (FDA) does not consider soap a cosmetic, it is not affected by the labeling laws requiring cosmetic ingredients to be listed, so most major manufacturers of soap do not give complete ingredient lists on soap labels.

The most popular and most heavily advertised soaps are the antimicrobial "deodorant" soaps. An FDA advisory review panel has questioned the safety of using these potent germ killers on a regular day-to-day, year-after-year basis. There is concern about possible dangerous consequences when these substances are absorbed through the skin and accumulate in the liver and other organs. As a result, the panel declared "not safe" or "not proved safe" those deodorant soaps containing **chloroxylenol, cloflucarban, phenol, triclocarban**, or **triclosan**. As I write this, the FDA is now taking action that will probably lead to a ban on triclosan—it's that toxic, and it's been in deodorant soap and many other products for years.

Despite all the advertising hoopla and questionable bactericides, the panel could find no evidence that these potentially hazardous substances actually helped stop body odor any more effectively than did plain soap!

In non-deodorant soaps, the most common and troublesome ingredient is synthetic fragrance. The fragrances in deodorant and luxury toilet soaps are clearly recognizable, but some of the other soaps commonly recognized as "pure" also contain added synthetic fragrance. Moreover, some soaps represented as "natural" contain synthetic fragrance (of, say, coconut or oatmeal) to enhance the scent of the natural ingredient. Not only are fragrances totally unnecessary to the cleaning effectiveness of soap, they are often irritating and can cause dry skin, redness, and rashes.

All you need is plain soap—no bactericides, no fragrances, no colors—just plain white soap.

Body odor is best prevented by regular bathing with plain soap and hot water. If you have a persistent, strong body odor problem, take it as a symptom that something is wrong with your body and see your health care professional. Healthy bodies smell sweet naturally.

Today there are many artisanal handmade soaps, made with natural ingredients that *are* listed on the label. And you can speak directly with the soap maker with any questions you have about ingredients. I usually see these soaps being sold by local soap makers at craft fairs and farmers' markets, and there are many online. You also can find plain soap at your natural-food store.

Remember, you can also make your own soap. It's not hard. Get a good soap-making book, and you may discover an enjoyable new hobby, or start a business.

Food

Food

The quality of the food you eat is intimately connected to your health. You might think of food as something that tastes good, something to socialize over, something that supplies nutrients, or something to watch celebrity chefs prepare on television, but food plays a vital role in your life, for the cells and organs of your body are literally made from the foods you eat. Your body health reflects the quality of the food you put into it. Toxic food results in a toxic body.

There are many toxic chemicals in our food supply.

Pesticides are the most toxic element in food. The EPA considers pesticides in food to be one of the nation's most serious health and environmental problems.

Pesticides used in agriculture have contaminated nearly all the air, water, soil, and living beings of the entire planet. According to an article in the *Des Moines Register*, the soil of America's bread basket is so saturated with pesticides that "our clouds are laced with pesticides . . . that have actually evaporated out of the ground along with the water, and rain down on us from the sky." Virtually all of us carry residues of toxic pesticides in the fat of our bodies.

Most food sold in supermarkets is sprayed heavily with pesticides, many of which cause cancer. We don't see warning labels on these foods that have been sprayed with pesticides, but they are on the containers of the pesticides. Here is the label for **malathion**, a pesticide commonly used on food crops:

KEEP OUT OF REACH OF CHILDREN. READ THE ENTIRE LABEL FIRST. OBSERVE ALL PRECAUTIONS AND FOLLOW DIRECTIONS CAREFULLY. HAZARDOUS TO HUMANS AND DOMESTIC ANIMALS. WARNING: Harmful if swallowed. Avoid breathing spray mists or vapors. Avoid contact with skin. Thoroughly wash after handling and before eating or smoking. Avoid contamination of feed and foodstuffs. Do not treat areas frequented by children and do not allow children in treated area until the spray has dried. Do not apply this product in such a manner as to directly or through drift expose workers or other persons. The area being treated must be vacated by unprotected persons.

Look at this: Thoroughly wash hands before eating. Avoid contamination of foodstuffs. Does it make sense to put this toxic substance in your body?

In addition to pesticide residues, fresh produce may be fumigated, irradiated, waxed, dyed with colors made from coal tar, and wrapped in papers containing fungicide. I remember the first time I tasted an organically grown orange that hadn't been shipped in a box. It tasted like an orange. It was only then that I realized the "flavor" I associated with fresh oranges was actually the fungicide from the shipping wrap.

Many more toxic chemicals are then used in food processing. In factories, foods are stripped of many of their nutrients as they are bleached, refined, colored, flavored, preserved, and packaged with attractive labels. Hundreds of food additives are used to make processed foods more appealing, and many of these additives are known to be harmful to health, including **sulfites, nitrates, artificial colors and flavors, MSG**, and **EDTA**. Most processed foods also contain **sugar** and **salt**, not in their natural forms, but refined into "pure" industrial chemicals that are harmful to health.

And then there are the toxic chemicals added to foods from packaging. Cans leach **bisphenol A** into their contents, adding a known endocrine disruptor to food. **Plastics** also migrate into foods from packaging.

These industrialized agribusiness foods can hardly be compared to the original foods provided by nature.

Research suggests that a primary contributing factor to many of our modern diseases is our eating of processed, low-fiber, low-nutrition foods. Before 1900, when most people ate foods simply prepared right from the farm, degenerative diseases were relatively rare. Today, cancer and heart disease cause half of all deaths. Obesity was a problem that generally affected only the wealthy, while today half our population is overweight to some degree.

Studies of other cultures that eat traditional, whole, unrefined, unprocessed foods show a remarkable lack of illness. And study after study has found that when people switch from their native diet to eating modern industrialized foods, they develop the diseases of the industrialized world.

HOW TO BE TOXIC-FREE

I know from my own experience how difficult it can be to change the way you eat. We all have our favorite foods, and food is closely tied to culture, family, and emotions. So I am going to give this to you step by step.

If you eat a lot of processed, packaged foods, just start reading labels and choose brands that do not have artificial colors and flavors, or preservatives. There are many, many brands to choose from now, sold even in major supermarkets and discount warehouses. Then look for packaged foods that are made with organically grown ingredients.

And then start learning to cook.

Ultimately, to be toxic-free, the goal is to prepare all your food at home from local, seasonal, organically grown ingredients.

Here's why this makes a difference.

In 2008, a Seattle newspaper reported a study conducted of the analysis of the urine and saliva of children eating a variety of conventional foods from local grocery stores. Biological markers of organophosphates, such as DDT and malathion, were present. When the same children ate organic fruits, vegetables, and juices, signs of pesticides were not found. The article stated:

> The transformation is extremely rapid. . . . Once you switch from conventional food to organic, the pesticides (malathion and chorphyifos) that we can measure in the urine disappears. The level returns immediately when you go back to the conventional diets.

Within eight to thirty-six hours of the children switching to organic food, the pesticides were no longer detected in the testing.

This, to me, is remarkable. When we eat organic food, we consume no toxic pesticides. When we don't eat organic food, we are literally eating poison.

Today there is more organically grown food available than ever before. You can find it:

* at your local natural-food store
* in many supermarkets (where I live here in Florida, the best place to buy organic poultry happens to be a big discount warehouse)
* at farmers' markets
* through Community Supported Agriculture (CSA; www.localharvest .org/csa) programs where you can buy direct from the farmer online

Start by just going shopping to look for organic food and see what is available. You don't need to change everything you eat all at once. Just buy one organic food that looks good to you and try it. Then buy another, and gradually switch over as you learn how to prepare fresh foods to your liking.

For more information on how to eat toxic-free, including choosing ingredients and delicious recipes, visit my website Toxic-Free Kitchen (www.toxicfreekitchen.com).

Coffee

Of all the foods and drinks, coffee is one of the most toxic. If you drink a cup of coffee every morning, and all you do is stop drinking toxic coffee, you will greatly reduce your toxic exposure.

Most coffee sold in the United States is grown in foreign countries that often use **pesticides** so toxic they have been banned here in this country.

The caffeine in coffee is responsible for many ills, including increased incidence of heart attacks, headaches, indigestion and ulcers, insomnia, anxiety, and depression. Pregnant women should limit their intake of caffeine; in large quantities it has contributed to the incidence of miscarriages, premature births, and birth defects.

Decaffeinated coffee contains residues of **hexane** and **methylene chloride** used in the decaffeinating process.

In addition, bleached white coffee filters may release trace amounts of **dioxin** into your cup of coffee. And if you drink it in a **polystyrene** cup, you're probably drinking a few molecules of plastic as well.

Instant gourmet flavored coffees may also contain **artificial flavors** and **sugar**.

On the other hand, coffee also has some health benefits *in moderation*. According to the Harvard Health Letter, coffee drinkers seem to have a lower risk for cancer and are less likely to develop diabetes.

I'm not going to tell you not to drink coffee, but I will recommend limiting your consumption of coffee and to avoid instant and flavored coffees.

Instead, use freshly ground coffee, preferably organically grown, and brew it using unbleached paper, cotton, or reusable metal coffee filters, or with a glass French press coffeemaker that self-filters the coffee grounds.

If you prefer decaffeinated coffee, drink steam- or water-processed varieties.

You might also try noncaffeinated hot beverages with flavors similar to coffee, such as those made from roasted grains (sold in natural-food stores).

And drink your coffee from a ceramic or glass mug.

I like drinking organically grown green tea, which you can purchase plain or blended with herbs and flowers in a variety of flavors. Fragrant and delicate, it seems to have a calming effect that at the same time provides a little pick-me-up. Green tea comes from the same leaves as black tea, but because it is not fermented, it retains its healthful ingredients, including significant amounts of vitamins and minerals. In Japan, green tea consumption goes up in winter, when fruits and fresh green vegetables are scarce. Medical researchers have discovered that green tea is effective in preventing some types of cancer and heart disease, helps regulate blood sugar levels, and provides other benefits.

Or drink any herbal tea that appeals to you—again, organically grown.

Remember that paper tea bags can contain a small amount of dioxin, too, so if you are going to drink tea, choose a brand with dioxin-free bags or, better yet, brew loose leaves. (I brew loose tea leaves in a French press coffeemaker, and it works wonderfully.)

Sweeteners

Sugar and other industrial sweeteners are ubiquitous throughout our food supply. Most processed foods contain some kind of sweetener, and sweeteners are not limited to desserts: salad dressings, barbecue sauce, sweet pickles, and other condiments usually contain sugar, as do bacon, ham, and other processed meats. Once I even found high-fructose corn syrup on the ingredients list of an egg salad sandwich on whole wheat bread!

If you want to reduce your toxic exposure in foods, eliminating refined sugar, high-fructose corn syrup, and artificial sweeteners should be at the top of your list.

Walk into any restaurant and every table will have a container with little packets of three colors. The pink packets are saccharin, the blue ones are aspartame, and the white are refined white sugar.

Saccharin (Sweet'N Low) is an artificial sweetener made in a laboratory from the by-products of crude-oil distillation. Though it is sweet, it is not a food, but it is popular because it has no calories and does not make blood sugar rise. For many years saccharin had a warning label that was required by law: "WARNING: Use of this product may be hazardous to your health. Contains saccharin, which has been determined to cause cancer in laboratory animals." Used as a sweetener since 1879, saccharin was accepted as safe until 1977, when a study done on rats found an excess of bladder cancers. In December 21, 2000, President Clinton signed a bill that removed the warning label. Studies do show that saccharin causes cancer in the urinary tract, bladder, lungs, ovaries, uterus, and other organs *in animals*. Officials who say it is safe claim that these animal studies are not relevant to humans, even though animal studies are the standard for identifying potential human carcinogens.

Aspartame (NutraSweet, Equal), another artificial sweetener that has no calories and produces no rise in blood sugar, is advertised as a "natural" sweetener made of the amino acids phenylalnine and aspartic acid, produced by growing bacteria. In your body, these naturally occurring substances break down into the same amino acids found in any protein food. Sounds harmless, but it isn't. Though the original amino acids from which aspartame is made exist in nature, the combination of them into aspartame does not: it is completely man-made, like any other industrial chemical. Large doses of phenylalanine are toxic to the brain and can contribute to headaches, depression, mood swings, high blood pressure, insomnia, and behavior problems. It can cause birth defects and is not recommended for use by pregnant women. Because aspartame is found in so many products—from soda to vitamin pills—it is easy to overdose without realizing it.

Refined white sugar is actually made from sugarcane or sugar beets, but by the time it is refined by industrial processes, it bears no resemblance to the natural whole food from which it comes. Most sugarcane and sugar beets have been sprayed with multiple pesticides, then processed over an open flame and chemically bleached. Refined white sugar has been associated with over 140 health problems, including nutritional deficiencies, lower resistance to disease, tooth decay, diabetes, hypoglycemia, heart disease, ulcers, and high blood pressure. It can stimulate your appetite, make you fat, and is as addictive as any drug (see the entire list at www.nancyappleton.com/141-reasons-sugar-ruins-your-health).

Sucralose (Splenda) is another artificial sweetener. Though it sounds good when advertisements say it is "made from sugar," what they don't tell you is that parts of the natural sugar molecule are replaced with chlorine. The jury is still out on the safety of sucralose. The manufacturer claims that the chlorine added to sucralose is similar to the chlorine atom in the salt (NaCl) molecule, but others say sucralose may be more like ingesting tiny amounts of chlorinated pesticides. By the time we find out, consumers may already be harmed. To me, the fact that there is such a thing as the Sucralose Toxicity Information Center (www.holisticmed.com/splenda) speaks volumes.

According to the definition of toxic, these sweeteners are all toxic chemicals that are negatively impacting your health.

HOW TO BE TOXIC-FREE

The first step is to simply buy unsweetened products—like unsweetened breakfast cereal—and add your own sweetener with discretion.

Then consider eating fewer sweet foods overall. Take a good look at what you are eating. Keep a journal for a week and write down everything you eat and just become aware of how much sugar, in all its many forms, you are putting in your body. If you are eating a lot of packaged processed foods—even if they are organic—you are getting a lot of sweeteners.

The solution, as difficult as this may sound, is to prepare your food at home, from whole organic ingredients, and add natural sweeteners in moderation. I know this will be a big change for you, but let me tell you, it is entirely worth doing.

For my entire life until about five years ago, I ate a lot of sugar in many different forms. But then I began to learn how even natural sweeteners were stressing my body, and I began to remove sweets from my diet. An amazing thing happened: I stopped craving sweets! My taste buds changed! Now even a bite of anything with refined white sugar tastes way too sweet to me. And my health improved.

I now mostly eat fruit when I want something sweet, and when I use a natural sweetener, I eat no more than a single teaspoonful. And that is plenty.

In recent years I have been intensively studying all the sweeteners sold in natural-food stores, and have come to the conclusion that the best natural sweeteners are those that are basically whole foods in their natural state or with their water removed.

The sweeteners I consider to be most healthy are:

- **raw organic honey:** a highly nutritious whole food in its natural state, produced by honeybees
- **organic evaporated cane juice:** the pressed juice of the sugarcane with the water removed, retaining the plant's nutrients
- **organic maple syrup and sugar:** the sap of the maple tree, boiled down to remove water

- **organic date sugar:** dehydrated dates ground into a powder
- **organic barley malt and brown rice syrups:** traditional Asian sweeteners made by sprouting and heating grains until the starch is turned to sugar
- **organic coconut or palm sugar:** my current favorite, made by boiling down the nectar of coconut blossoms and grinding the resulting powder into fine crystals

New whole-food sweeteners, which I am still experimenting with, continue to come onto the market; they include Jerusalem artichoke syrup, yacón syrup, lúcuma powder, and others.

Most of these sweeteners can be purchased at your local natural-food store. All can be purchased on the Internet.

I don't recommend so-called natural sweeteners xylitol and stevia because the form in which they are sold is so highly refined, they are no longer whole foods. I do grow stevia as an herb in my garden and pick the leaves to brew with my tea for calorie-free sweetness. I also at the moment don't recommend agave, as much as I like it, because there is controversy over how it is produced, how refined it is, and how it might affect your body. I may change my mind as I get more documented information.

I am frequently asked "What is the best . . . ?" and "What is the healthiest . . . ?" As with other products, there isn't a sweetener that is best for all. Each body has different needs. One person may choose a low-glycemic sweetener to control their blood sugar, while another person who has normal blood sugar may prefer honey because it is natural and flavorful and has life-enhancing properties.

Whichever sweetener you choose, eat it in moderation as part of a well-balanced diet. Even if these sweeteners are natural or organically grown, that doesn't mean they are nutritious foods. Use them sparingly.

For more information on natural sweeteners and how to use them, visit my website Sweet Savvy (www.sweetsavvy.com).

Vitamin and Mineral Dietary Supplements

In today's world, the reality is that most people need to take dietary supplements. Even if you eat a balanced diet of whole organic foods, your body needs more nutrients than foods can provide to combat the levels of stress and toxic exposure that are common (more about this in Chapter 4).

But you don't want to take the heavily advertised, brightly colored, high-potency multivitamins with clever names. They generally contain **artificial colors**, **artificial flavors**, the preservatives **BHA** and **BHT**, **mineral oil**, **sugar**, **sulfites**, and **talc**. The brightly colored coatings may be made from plastic; those in gelatin capsules are usually preserved with **formaldehyde** unless otherwise stated.

And the vitamins themselves are made in laboratories from crude oil.

HOW TO BE TOXIC-FREE

As a first step, at least take supplements that are additive-free. Your local natural-food store is full of them, so you should have no problem finding them.

The next question is whether you should take vitamins and minerals made from natural sources or synthetic vitamins made from petrochemicals.

Even though many people claim that natural and synthetic supplements are chemically identical, natural supplements do have molecular, biological, and electromagnetic differences that produce greater levels of biological activity and are therefore better utilized by the body than synthetic forms.

In some cases, synthetic vitamins have entirely different chemical structures than their natural counterparts found in food. In their book *The Body Electric: Electromagnetism and the Foundation of Life*, Robert O. Becker, M.D., and Gary Selden state:

All organic compounds . . . are identified by the way they bend light in solution. The dextrorotatory (D) forms rotate it to the right, while levorotatory (L) isomers refract it to the left. All artificial methods of synthesizing organic compounds yield roughly equal mixtures of D and L molecules. However, living things consist of *either* D *or* L forms, depending on the species, but *never both.*

Most of the thousands of vitamin products on the market obtain their raw ingredients from three *pharmaceutical* companies, all based in Europe. Most so-called natural vitamins on the market today are either fortified (a very small amount of low-potency natural vitamins mixed with high-potency synthetic vitamins) or are synthetic vitamins in a very small amount of natural base (the label will say something like "in a natural base containing . . .").

The only true natural vitamins are those that come from organic foods. They are available in nutritional supplements as highly nutritious, concentrated foods; powdered concentrates of foods and herbs with the moisture removed; and an isolated component of a food. (Read more in Chapter 4: Take Organic Whole-Food Supplements on page 149.)

Organic food-source supplements are more widely available today than ever before—even from mass-market retailers. So look for them.

Cookware

POTS AND PANS with "non-stick" finishes made with PFOAs—also known as Teflon, Silverstone, and other trade names—should not be used, period. At the moment, perfluorooctanoic acid (PFOA) is not fully understood, but there is sufficient concern from animal studies that the EPA is investigating it. There is concern because PFOA is found throughout the environment and in the blood of the general U.S. population, and it is very persistent in the environment and in bodies. In my opinion, the precautionary principle (see page 227) should be applied here, especially since there is toxic-free non-stick cookware.

Aluminum cookware should not be used if the cooking surface comes in contact with the food. Foods cooked in aluminum can react with the metal to form aluminum salts. Little research has been done on the amount of exposure we may receive from food cooked in aluminum cookware or its health effects, but aluminum salts from other sources of exposure have been connected with brain disorders such as dementia, Alzheimer's disease, behavior abnormalities, poor memory, and impaired motor-visual coordination. One British study showed that foods cooked in aluminum cookware may cause indigestion, heartburn, intestinal gas, constipation, and headaches. And a study in Sri Lanka showed that the amount of aluminum that leaches into food increases one thousand times when fluoridated water is used for cooking.

Stainless steel cookware (or copper cookware lined with stainless steel) may also be harmful. Here the problem is scratching the surface. When using metal utensils, scratching the surface can "open" the metal, allowing small amounts of highly toxic meals such as chromium and nickel to be released into food. When exposed to air, however, the stainless steel "heals" the "wound," once again sealing the metals into the alloy. But if you use metal utensils on metal cookware, each time you open the possibility of heavy metals getting into your food.

HOW TO BE TOXIC-FREE

We need not use cookware with suspected toxic non-stick finishes because there are now a number of cookware brands that have PFOA-free non-stick finishes. There appear to me to be two types: one is a PFOA plastic, which is still a plastic of some sort, and the other is a very slippery ceramic, which I prefer.

The safe cookwares are:

- **glass**
- **cast iron**

- **porcelain enamel-coated cast iron or stainless steel**
- **terra-cotta clay** (check to make sure the glaze doesn't contain lead, particularly if the item is imported)
- **ceramic** (this is high-tech ceramic through and through)

Cookware made from all of these materials is available at most department stores, home warehouse stores, and kitchen shops, and on the Internet.

Anodized aluminum is another possible choice. Aluminum is a favored metal for cookware because it distributes heat evenly. Though there are health problems associated with aluminum cookware, if a label says the cookware is made from *anodized* aluminum, it is safe to use. This means that the aluminum was dipped into a hot acid bath that seals the aluminum by changing its molecular structure. Once anodized, the aluminum will not leach into the food.

Dishware and Glassware

Prop 65 Warning: This product contains lead, a chemical known to the State of California to cause cancer, birth defects, and other reproductive harm.

THE HIDDEN danger in ceramic dishware is the **lead** used in glazes. And it's not just brightly colored dishware from other countries that is the problem: most major manufacturers of dinnerware sold in department stores and home-decorating shops still use lead glazes without labeling them as such.

The federal government prohibits the sale of dinnerware that releases lead in amounts greater than 2,000 ppb (which prevents direct cases of lead poisoning), but the state of California requires warning labels on any dishware that releases lead in amounts greater than 224 ppb, to protect against long-term health risks. But that's not enough in my book. There is no safe level for lead exposure.

If you don't live in the state of California and therefore don't have warning labels on dishware that contains lead, ask the salesperson before you buy to verify with the manufacturer whether or not a lead-free glaze was used on the particular pattern you are interested in. Often local potters use lead-free glazes and with them you have the advantage of being able to ask the person who actually made the dish what kind of glaze was used.

You can also purchase clear glass dishware or wooden plates and bowls, which have no glaze at all.

If you have dishware that you suspect may have a lead finish, you can test it with a home lead-testing kit.

Food Storage

The toxic concern for food storage is plastic, obviously, as most food storage containers are made of plastic.

Though food storage containers, bags, and wraps usually just say "plastic" in big letters on the label, if you look closer at the fine print, it will often say what type of plastic it is made from. If not, contact the manufacturer to find out.

What you want to watch out for are food storage products made from **polyvinyl chloride (PVC)**, which leaches phthalates, a known endocrine disruptor, or **bisphenol A (BPA)**, also an endocrine disruptor.

These toxic plastics can migrate into food that is stored in them for any length of time.

HOW TO BE TOXIC-FREE

The very best option for storing food is glass. Glass jars and containers come in a variety of sizes. If you don't find them locally, there are websites where you can order almost any size and shape for very little money. If you want to freeze food in glass containers, use canning jars that come in boxes labeled "for canning and freezing" and leave space for food or liquid to expand. Regular glass containers may crack as food expands during freezing.

But I also understand that sometimes using glass can be unrealistic. If you do need to use plastic, choose food storage products made from polypropylene, which has a very low toxicity. The "disposable" storage containers are made from polypropylene and can be reused many times.

For maximum safety, do not microwave food in plastic containers, place hot food in plastic containers, or feed your baby warm formula in plastic baby bottles. Heat makes plastic migrate from container into food or liquid. And whether the health effects of a particular plastic are yet known or not, plastic is not natural to your body.

Textiles
Clothing

Clothing for men, women, and children is made from a wide variety of fabrics that contain chemicals of varying toxicity.

First, the fabrics used to make most clothing today are made from synthetic fibers that are actually plastics made from petrochemicals: **nylon**, **polyester**, and **acrylic** are among the more popular. Very little research has been done on the possible toxic effects of wearing plastic fibers. Yet, they continuously give off minute plastic vapors as the plastic is warmed against your skin. And they require toxic chemicals to maintain them—chemicals such as synthetic detergents and fabric softeners with neurotoxic **artificial scents** to reduce static cling.

But more toxic are the fabric finishes. All polyester/cotton and permanent-press cotton clothing is coated with a resin that releases vapors of **formaldehyde** (see Bedsheets, page 94).

Choose clothing made from natural fibers: cotton, linen, silk, all the various types of wool, or ramie.

A second choice would be rayon, lyocell, or bamboo. These are man-made fibers composed of cellulose, a substance found in all plants. The cellulose used to make rayon is recycled cotton linters, old cotton rags, paper, and wood pulp. Lyocell is a cellulosic fiber made from wood. The fabric sold as "bamboo" is also a man-made cellulosic fiber, using quick-growing bamboo as the cellulose material. Though these fibers begin as natural materials, they are not in their natural state, as are cotton, linen, silk, and wool.

Today there is more and more clothing available from untreated. organically grown, naturally dyed natural fiber fabrics than ever before, as the fashion industry has taken an interest in going green. If you don't find what you are looking for locally, look online.

It's a good idea to wash any clothing before you wear it to remove any finishes or residues that may be on the fabric.

Bedsheets

POISON! DANGER! SUSPECT CANCER HAZARD. MAY CAUSE CANCER. Risk of cancer depends on level and duration of exposure. VAPOR HARMFUL. HARMFUL IF INHALED OR ABSORBED THROUGH SKIN. CAUSES IRRITATION TO SKIN, EYES AND RESPIRATORY TRACT. STRONG SENSITIZER. MAY BE FATAL OR CAUSE BLINDNESS IF SWALLOWED. CANNOT BE MADE NONPOISONOUS. FLAMMABLE LIQUID AND VAPOR.

IF YOU are taking sleeping pills or other sleep aids for insomnia, you may not need them. The problem may be your bedsheets.

All polyester/cotton and permanent-press cotton bedsheets are coated with a resin that releases vapors of **formaldehyde**, and formaldehyde causes insomnia. Yes, the sheets you are sleeping on may be keeping you awake at night. While all polyester/cotton fabrics have formaldehyde finishes, bedsheets have a particularly heavy finish because of their continuous use and frequent laundering. The finishing process combines formaldehyde resin directly with the fiber, making it impossible to remove, yet it emits formaldehyde vapors night after night in your bed.

Formaldehyde has also been classified as a substance known to cause cancer in humans by the International Agency for Research on Cancer. The warning label above is off a bottle of formaldehyde.

The National Academy of Sciences estimates that 10 to 20 percent of the general population may be susceptible to the irritant properties of formaldehyde at extremely low concentrations.

Other symptoms of formaldehyde exposure include coughing, swelling of the throat, watery eyes, respiratory problems, tiredness, and more.

It's time to change your sheets.

It's also a good idea to wash any sheets before you put them on your bed to remove any finishes or residues that may be on the fabric.

HOW TO BE TOXIC-FREE

Go shopping and buy a new set of sheets and pillowcases that are not treated with a no-iron finish. Most department and large houseware stores now sell them.

Choose any cotton flannel or cotton knit sheets, or woven cotton sheets that are labeled "untreated" or "formaldehyde-free."

Bed linens made from organically grown cotton are now widely available and affordable too. Most do not have permanent-press finishes, but check the label to be sure.

You don't have to iron cotton sheets. Just pull them out of the dryer the minute the dryer cycle ends. Wrinkles are created when the hot fabric sits in a crumpled mess. Remove your sheets from the dryer and fold them, or put them right on the bed, and you won't need to iron. Flannel and knit sheets don't wrinkle at all.

After you change your sheets, you may also want to consider a natural-fiber pillow and a natural-fiber comforter or blankets. And when you're ready to make an investment, a natural-fiber mattress.

Shoes

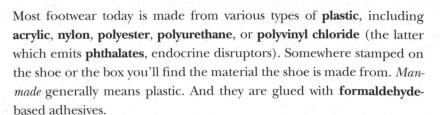

Most footwear today is made from various types of **plastic**, including **acrylic, nylon, polyester, polyurethane**, or **polyvinyl chloride** (the latter which emits **phthalates**, endocrine disruptors). Somewhere stamped on the shoe or the box you'll find the material the shoe is made from. *Man-made* generally means plastic. And they are glued with **formaldehyde**-based adhesives.

One of the more recent additions to the list of toxic chemicals found in shoes is **antimicrobials**, added to kill bacteria and fungus and prevent odors. Generally, shoe manufacturers are reluctant to disclose what the antimicrobial is; however, I learned from a chemist it is often **triclosan**, another endocrine disruptor. In 2010, the FDA and EPA stated they were taking another look at triclosan, as recent research has raised "valid concerns" about its safety.

Socks and stockings are also made from plastics, generally acrylic or nylon.

And watch out for shoes made from recycled plastic or recycled rubber tires. Though recycling is better for the environment, it does not reduce the toxicity of the plastic or synthetic rubber used to make tires.

HOW TO BE TOXIC-FREE

First, if you wear socks (I say this because here in Florida I wear sandals on my bare feet almost every day of the year), wear cotton socks rather than plastics. They are much softer than the plastic fibers and absorb moisture better, making them much more comfortable. If you can't find cotton socks in a local store, you can order them on the Internet.

As with many other products, there are more toxic-free shoes available than ever before. A number of brands are made from natural materials, including leather, cotton, and hemp. They can be found in natural-shoe boutiques, in department stores, and online. And stay away from any shoes that contain unknown antibacterials.

Look for leather shoes that are "naturally processed" or "vegetable-tanned" to avoid toxic agents used in leather processing. Some shoes made from leather may emit fumes from tanning when you first buy them, but they are volatile and will dissipate if you leave the shoes outdoors for a few days. And if you wear a type of leather shoe that requires shoe polish, you can buy shoe polish made from natural ingredients online.

A new material being used to make shoes as an alternative to polyvinyl chloride is EVA, which is ethylene vinyl acetate, a copolymer of ethylene and vinyl acetate. Like PVC, EVA is made from petrochemicals, but it has very low toxicity.

Irons and Ironing-Board Covers

Okay, let's face it: if you are going to wear natural fibers, you are just going to have to do a certain amount of ironing. So you'll want ironing to be a safe experience too.

Nowadays, most irons and ironing board covers are coated with **tetrafluoroethylene** plastic, better known as Teflon. Given that heating plastic makes it outgas its toxic fumes, irons and ironing-board covers seem odd places to put it, particularly since a non-stick finish is not even necessary for the task. Tetrafluoroethylene fumes can be irritating to eyes, nose, and throat, and can cause breathing difficulties.

HOW TO BE TOXIC-FREE

First, minimize your need to iron by removing clothing from the dryer the moment the cycle finishes. I've even been known to toss something in the dryer to remove wrinkles rather than iron: it works great. All you need is a few minutes.

Second, choose clothing that doesn't require ironing. I live in Florida and wear cotton virtually every day. Most of the year I wear cotton drawstring capri pants with a cotton knit tank top. I have one drawer for pants and one drawer for tank tops. I never need to iron either.

But occasionally I do dress up, and then I need to iron. Cover your ironing board with a plain cotton pad and cover. These are sold in every good hardware store and online. Then get yourself a good iron, not a cheap one. I have one with a shiny heating surface (no Teflon), and I was surprised the first time I used it what a difference a good iron makes. It's heavy to lift, but it glides along the fabric so smoothly, removing every wrinkle without any pressure on my part.

Yes, it can be drudgery to iron, but the pleasure and health I gain from the natural fibers is more than worth whatever time and effort it takes to maintain them.

Interior Decorating
Wall Paint

  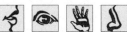

Warning: Harmful or fatal if swallowed. May cause slight skin irritation and eye irritation. Vapor and spray mist may be harmful if inhaled.

Caution: Use with adequate ventilation. Where ventilation is inadequate, use a suitable respirator. In case of eye contact, flush eyes immediately with plenty of water for at least 15 minutes. Do not take internally. Keep out of reach of children.

ALL PAINT is made from four categories of ingredients:

- **resins** for adhesion and durability
- **pigments** for color and covering power
- **additives** to enhance performance properties
- **solvents** (usually the largest component found in paint), which serve as carriers to dissolve and disperse the other ingredients

Paints are generally classified according to the type of solvent they contain: oil-based paints contain **volatile organic chemical (VOC)** solvents (40 to 60 percent), and water-based paints use water as the primary solvent (though they still generally contain 5 to 10 percent VOC solvents).

Oil-based paints contain **ethylbenzene**, various **butyl ethers**, **mineral spirits**, and **xylene**. Collectively they affect your central nervous system and can cause dizziness, headaches, tightening of the chest, breathing difficulties, vomiting, and irritation of the eyes, nose, throat, and skin. Water-based paints, on the other hand, contain only the butyl ethers. Wood finishes contain similar solvents.

In the Los Angeles basin, famous for its smog, it was found that VOCs from paints released more VOCs than all of the region's oil refineries and gas stations *combined*. Southern California now has the strictest VOC regulations for paints in the country.

A Johns Hopkins University study found that more than 300 toxic chemicals and 150 carcinogens may be present in paint, depending on the individual formula. They include **aerosol propellants**, **ammonia**, **benzene**, **ethanol**, **formaldehyde**, **glycols**, **kerosene**, **lead**, **pentachlorophenol**, **phenol**, **plastics** (**acrylonitrile**, **latex**, **phenolformaldehyde resin**, **polyester**, **polyurethane**, **tetrafluoroethylene**), **toluene**, **trichloroethylene**, and **xylene**.

HOW TO BE TOXIC-FREE

Because of concerns about the effects of VOCs on outdoor air pollution, most oil-based paints are being phased out and new, much less toxic paints are being introduced.

All the major paint manufacturers now make less toxic paints. These are called low-VOC or no-VOC paints. Ask for them specifically where you purchase paint. They are now sold even in major home improvement stores.

Three German companies sell paints in America made from plant-based ingredients. Their common philosophy is to use ingredients produced from nature, which nature can replenish and will return to nature, and are safe for the user's health. Two of the brands contain nontoxic petrochemical solvents, and the third uses a renewable balsam **terpene** solvent that is considered in Europe to be of questionable safety. Still, they are safer for health and the environment than petrochemical-based paints. I have used these paints, and even though they give beautiful finishes, there is one drawback: the plant oils and resins have *very* strong odors. Not toxic, but strong.

Then there are paints of a completely different sort. Milk paint is a casein-based paint that is great for furniture, wood, and walls. It comes in powder form, and you mix it up. It's what everyone used before we had plastic paints (available online).

When I remodeled my bathroom a few years ago, I used colored clay plaster on the walls instead of paint. It was easy to apply and looks beautiful.

Carpeting

SYNTHETIC CARPETING is made from a complex blend of materials that can emit as many as 120 hazardous chemicals. They include **pesticides** (such as **antimicrobials**), **neurotoxic solvents** (such as **toluene** and **xylene**), and the potent carcinogen **benzene**. **Formaldehyde** is also commonly emitted from carpets, according to reports by the EPA and the Consumer Product Safety Commission.

The danger of toxic chemicals in carpets was headline news back in 1988, when more than 10 percent of employees at the offices of the EPA reported symptoms after exposure to new carpeting. These were as diverse as burning eyes, memory problems, chills and fever, sore throats, joint pain, coughing, numbness, nausea, dizziness, blurred vision, nervousness, depression, and difficulty concentrating.

As a result of the investigations that followed this incident, the EPA determined that synthetic carpeting is a major contributor to indoor air pollution.

HOW TO BE TOXIC-FREE

In response to concerns about carpet's contribution to indoor air quality, the carpet industry, through the Carpet and Rug Institute, responded with the CRI Green Label (www.carpet-rug.org/residential-customers/selecting-the-right-carpet-or-rug/green-label.cfm). Independent laboratory tests identify low-emitting carpeting, adhesives, and cushion materials that meet scientifically established standards. Products that meet these standards are allowed to display the logo.

Since the program began in 1992, carpet manufacturers have made substantial reductions in the levels of chemicals that outgas from carpets.

If you must have a carpet, choose one from the CRI Green Label program, or one made from natural fibers.

However, my best recommendation for toxic-free flooring is to eliminate wall-to-wall carpets altogether.

Solid-wood hardwood flooring is one of the safest floorings you can have in your home. In addition to its warmth and beauty, wood itself is completely toxic-free and a renewable resource. I generally recommend installing prefinished flooring, which comes with a baked-on finish. Be sure to choose a solid wood floor, not laminate, and not engineered, which often are glued together with adhesives that emit **formaldehyde** and other chemicals.

Natural linoleum is another good choice. Made from linseed oil, pine tree resins, wood flour from deciduous trees, and cork, which are mixed with chalk, clay, and colored mineral pigments, then put on a jute backing, it provides an attractive and durable floor covering. Dealers who sell natural linoleum also sell safe adhesives for installation.

Cork tiles also are becoming popular as a natural floor covering. Durable and economical, cork is warm underfoot and provides noise insulation while looking rich and beautiful. In the 1920s, Frank Lloyd

Wright chose cork as a finishing material in the natural homes he designed, and it has been popular ever since.

You can also use ceramic tile, brick, marble and other stone tiles, cement, or terrazzo.

Furniture

MOST HOME furnishings are made from materials that give off toxic fumes.

Bookcases and desks are often made from particleboard and plywood, which outgas **formaldehyde**, an irritant to eyes, nose, and throat and a suspected carcinogen.

Pillows and padding on stuffed sofas and chairs are generally made from **polyurethane** foam plastic and can be covered with **acrylic**, **polyester**, or **polyvinyl chloride** plastic covers. Most upholstery fabrics are covered with a formaldehyde resin to resist stains. One study showed that the addition of furniture to an otherwise empty room tripled formaldehyde levels.

HOW TO BE TOXIC-FREE

As much as possible, purchase furniture made from natural materials. This doesn't have to be expensive, as many pieces can be purchased used.

My desk, where I am sitting while writing this book, is a big old oak library table from the Stanford University library that I bought at a salvage store for twenty-five dollars. The edges were worn, but I had them sawed off, sanded them down, and trimmed the whole table with purpleheart wood, which, yes, is purple! Then I had it finished with several coats of water-based wood finish.

Upholstered furniture should be covered with a prewashed natural-fiber fabric and stuffed with cotton or wool batting or feathers. I bought my sofa at an auction for fifty dollars. It's a beautiful old sofa with wood arms and a nice curve in the back. I had the spring-filled cushions refurbished with new cotton and the whole thing covered with untreated linen upholstery fabric. That was years ago and it still looks like new.

My dining table was another garage-sale find—another solid-oak library table that didn't even need refinishing. Around it are four Shaker chairs that I built from kits. I applied my own toxic-free finish to the wood pieces and wove the cotton webbing seats together with a friend (it really is a two-person job). Not only are these chairs toxic-free, they are also beautiful and I often experience the satisfaction of our my workmanship.

I also purchase furniture from unfinished-wood-furniture stores and apply my own toxic-free water-based wood finishes. When purchasing solid-wood furniture, check carefully to make sure that it is indeed *solid* wood. Often the front will be wood and the backs, sides, inside shelves, and drawer bottoms will be particleboard or plywood. Particleboard can be very convincingly veneered, but veneer poses no barrier to formaldehyde emissions.

Candles

THERE ARE no warning labels on candles because candle manufacturers are not required by law to list or disclose hazardous, toxic, or carcinogenic compounds used as ingredients in their products. But that does not mean there are not toxic chemicals present.

Most candles, unless otherwise labeled, are made from paraffin, a by-product of the gasoline industry. They produce the same combustion by-products as any other burning petrochemical (see Carbon Monoxide, on page 41), though in a lesser amount. Fumes from the paraffin wax itself have been found to cause kidney and bladder tumors in laboratory animals.

Some paraffin candles still have lead core wicks. According to preliminary tests, particles of **lead** do volatilize during normal candle burning. Simply breathing in small particulate matter can irritate and damage the lungs, causing breathing problems, in particular affecting those with asthma or some type of lung or heart disease. But even worse, preliminary wipe test results show 40 milligrams of lead per square foot in a home that burned a number of lead core wick candles, an astounding amount for a substance for which there is no safe level. One hundred percent of lead that is inhaled is absorbed into the bloodstream.

Scented candles contain even more toxics. Candlemakers are using increasing amounts of (often artificial) fragrance oils in their wax mixtures—some of which are not even suitable for combustion. Toxic chemicals that have been found in the combustion by-products of some scented candles include **acetone, benzene, carbon tetrachloride, trichloroethene, toluene, styrene, xylene, phenol, cresol, lead, carbon monoxide,** and other toxic substances as well as particulate matter.

But gel candles are the worst. These are made from specially processed petrochemical mineral oils gelled with plastic polymers, poured into glass containers. You can recognize gel candles by the clearness of the gel (which is often colored), the rubbery texture, and the glass container, and they often have "embeds" in them. Most gel candles are also scented with artificial fragrances, some highly so. Because gel candles are made from the same petrochemicals and fragrances used to make paraffin candles, the hazards of burning them are similar. However, the greatest danger is that candles that are improperly made or have glass containers that are too thin tend to explode, blowing shattered glass all over the room and anyone that is nearby. These exploding candles have even been known to set houses on fire.

HOW TO BE TOXIC-FREE

Burn beeswax candles with cotton wicks. Their natural sweet honey fragrance is delicious. There are two types: solid, which are dipped or molded, and rolled, which are made from thin sheets of beeswax stamped with a honeycomb pattern. Some of the molded beeswax candles have hollow centers. The rolled and hollow candles do not burn very long, but the solid ones burn very well. These are available in some candle stores and most natural-food stores, as well as on the Internet.

Beeswax candles are often bleached or tinted with artificial colors, so look for those that are their natural deep-honey color. Beeswax candles are more expensive than paraffin candles; to reduce the price, you can purchase sheets of beeswax at most craft stores and easily roll your own.

For the holidays, try bayberry candles. A New England tradition, they are made from bayberries, which are boiled in water to release their wax. According to legend, the burning of bayberry candles during the holiday season brings wealth and good luck to the household. Look for them made by a local candle maker, in gift shops and catalogs from New England, and on the Internet. Be sure to check that the candle itself is made from the wax of the bayberry plant, not just "bayberry scented."

"Soy wax" candles are made primarily from soybean oil. Some candles are 100 percent soy; others are made from 90 percent soy oil mixed with other plant ingredients such as corn and carnauba. Soy candles burn extremely clean and do not give off the oily soot that can leave a residue on walls and furniture and aggravate asthma and other breathing problems. Soy candles will also burn about 25 percent longer than similar paraffin candles. Because the makers of soy candles are often motivated by their concern for health, they generally use other natural ingredients as well, such as high-quality natural essential oils for fragrance and lead free, unbleached cotton wicks. Soy candles are sold in gift shops, natural-food stores, and on the Internet.

If you want to burn scented candles, make sure they are authentic aromatherapy candles that are scented with real essential oils. If the label isn't clear about this, call the manufacturer before purchasing.

Lightbulbs

 LAMP CONTAINS MERCURY. Manage in accordance with disposal laws.

IN PAST BOOKS, I've written about how artificial light produced by light-bulbs—fluorescents in particular—can be hazardous to health. This is still true.

The problem with artificial light sources seems to be that the spectrum of the light produced is not the same as the spectrum produced by natural sunlight. Our bodies need the natural light of the sun, and tend to function somewhat less than optimally when we spend most of our hours under unnatural light.

Exposure to artificial light has been associated with osteoporosis, dental caries, fatigue, decreased sharpness of vision, hyperactivity, and changes in heart rate, blood pressure, electrical brain-wave patterns, hormonal secretions, and the body's cyclical rhythms.

But now the widespread use of compact fluorescent lightbulbs compel me to write about the toxic danger of lightbulbs.

All fluorescent bulbs contain mercury. They all have warning labels that the lamp contains mercury; this warning is for proper disposal, but not to alert consumers about toxic danger.

According to the EPA, "Exposure to mercury, a toxic metal, can affect our brain, spinal cord, kidneys and liver, causing symptoms such as trembling hands, memory loss, and difficulty moving." So the warning label *should* be for health as well.

The EPA also says, "Mercury is released into our environment when products with mercury are broken, disposed of improperly, or incinerated. If you break a CFL, clean it up safely."

If you think that your compact fluorescent bulbs are safe from breakage, let me tell you of my experience. A reader wrote to me "scared to death" because her daughter had accidentally knocked over a lamp and broken the compact fluorescent bulb. And I once observed with my own eyes a mother drop a compact fluorescent bulb on her way to replacing a burned-out bulb, and then she just wiped it up with her bare hands and a paper towel and put it in the trash. Breakage happens. And when it does, you contaminate your home with mercury.

Though the Material Safety Data Sheet says that there is no harm from the amount of mercury you would be exposed to from a broken bulb, the EPA gives extensive directions on how to clean up a broken compact fluorescent bulb and dispose of it. It includes removing people and pets from the room, shutting off central forced-air HVAC systems, and placing the broken pieces in a sealable container.

For more information, see Frequently Asked Questions: Information on Compact Fluorescent Bulbs (CFLs) and Mercury (www.energy star.gov/ia/partners/promotions/change_light/downloads/Fact _Sheet_Mercury.pdf).

HOW TO BE TOXIC-FREE

The hot new lighting technology is light-emitting diodes (LEDs). These bulbs consume dramatically less power, convert energy to light (not heat), and have an extremely long life (50,000 hours!).

The one drawback is that LEDs—like compact fluorescents—contain toxics (**lead** and **arsenic**), but the danger is much less than with compact fluorescent bulbs. LEDs are virtually indestructible, so there is little chance you will be exposed to these metals at home, and even when LEDs go to the landfill and are crushed, the amount of toxic metals contained within them that might spread into the environment is much less, and the bulbs can be easily recycled when programs are set up to do so. LEDs can now be found in many spectrum shades, from cool to warm to natural white, which is just like sunlight, at most hardware and home improvement stores.

I also save energy by using task lights in most rooms rather than overhead lights. In my office, I have only one small desk lamp and seventeen feet of picture windows. In the kitchen, I have a track of halogens right over the sink with a separate switch that illuminates just the work area, in addition to the overhead room light. In the bedroom, I have only two small reading lamps. In the bathroom I have a large skylight. So I reduce air pollution and save energy by using less artificial light as well as using energy-saving lightbulbs.

If you do choose to use tube or compact fluorescent bulbs, be sure to recycle them to keep mercury from going into the environment. You can take them to any Home Depot for recycling or recycle them through www.lamprecycle.org or www.lamprecycling.com.

Home Office
Permanent Markers

EVEN THOUGH there are no warning labels, markers that have "permanent" ink contain very toxic volatile solvents, including neurotoxicants **toluene** and **xylene**.

Toluene is so dangerous that it is included on the EPA's list of 129 "priority pollutants" recognized as being hazardous to human health. Toluene primarily affects the mind and nervous system, causing depression, irritability, and disorientation.

Exposure to xylene can cause dizziness, feelings of euphoria, giddiness, and headaches, as well as confusion, coma, and death.

There's just no need to be exposed to chemicals that do this degree of harm to our bodies when there are safe alternatives easily available.

HOW TO BE TOXIC-FREE

Check through your markers and throw away any with "permanent" ink.

Get some color in your life without toxic solvents by choosing water-based markers.

Water-based markers for children are available anywhere markers are sold. Look for the word *washable* on the label.

If you are an artist and want a wider variety of colors, go to a good art supply store. There you will find water-based markers with many different tip widths, and even brush tips.

It's easy to tell which markers contain solvents and which are water-based by smelling them. The solvent-based markers have a strong odor, while the water-based markers smell like nothing. It's very obvious.

Also, check with your child's day care or school to see if they use permanent-ink markers. Fumes from these markers certainly *don't* help a child to think and learn.

Epoxy, Rubber Cement, and Super Glue

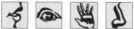

Danger: Extremely flammable. Vapor harmful. Harmful or fatal if swallowed. Skin and eye irritant. Keep out of reach of children. Bonds skin instantly. Toxic.

Caution: Do not use near sparks or flame. Do not breathe vapors. Use in well-ventilated room. Keep away from small children.

ADHESIVES ARE full of volatile chemicals. **Naphthalene, phenol, ethanol, vinyl chloride, formaldehyde, acrylonitrile,** and **epoxy** are a few of the chemicals more commonly used. All these substances release toxic vapors.

Although you probably wouldn't die from the amount of vapors you would breathe in during normal use of an adhesive, these adhesives are widely misused to get high. According to the National Inhalant Prevention Coalition, inhaling dangerous products is becoming one of the most widespread problems in the United States.

Nearly all abused inhalants produce slowed-down body functions. Depending upon the amount inhaled, the user can experience slight stimulation, feeling of less inhibition, or loss of consciousness, and can even die. The most significant toxic effect of chronic exposure to inhalants is widespread and long-lasting damage to the brain and other parts of the nervous system. Similar effects could occur if you use solvent-based adhesives regularly without adequate ventilation.

Other common household products that are often used for inhalant abuse include shoe polish, gasoline, lighter fluid, spray paint, correction fluid, cleaning fluid, and paint thinner.

HOW TO BE TOXIC-FREE

There are plenty of toxic-free glues available that are appropriate for household use.

The safest glues on the market are white glues and yellow woodworking glues, both widely available at most stores. White glue effectively bonds paper, cloth, wood, pottery, and most other porous and semiporous materials. It is quick-drying, clear, and nontoxic. I've even been known to use it to lay hardwood floors (worked great!).

For gluing paper, try a glue stick. This is the household glue I use the most. These are solid, very-low-odor white glues.

I've also discovered a clear liquid nontoxic glue in a squeeze bottle. The brand I bought had the word *nontoxic* and the Certified Product logo of the Art & Creative Materials Institute.

If a toxic adhesive is the *only* glue that will do the job, use it in a well-ventilated area (outdoors is best) and wear a protective mask and gloves. Once completely dry, the adhesives are safe, but you'll want to protect yourself well during application.

CHAPTER 3

Environment

For the first time in the history of the world, every human being is now subjected to contact with dangerous chemicals, from the moment of conception until death.

—RACHEL CARSON
Silent Spring (1962)

S INCE THIS is a book about how toxic chemicals can make you sick and what you can do to get well, why is there a chapter about the environment?

Because toxic chemicals in the environment are damaging the environment itself, polluting the air, water, and soil that sustain ecosystems, and altering or killing many species. And even though we spend 90 percent of our time indoors, we are still exposed to enough polluted air, water, and soil in the environment for them to be sources of toxic chemical exposures that can damage the health of our bodies.

For me, the environment isn't "out there" somewhere. I live in it, and what I do to it—for better or worse—directly affects my own health and well-being. Without the earth, we would have no air to breathe or food to eat or houses to live in. So, for me, the health of our bodies is completely dependent on the environment. It's all one system of life.

We must safeguard and protect the environment at large in order to safeguard and protect our own bodies.

We need look no further than Rachel Carson's groundbreaking book *Silent Spring* for evidence that the earth is contaminated with toxic chemicals that are damaging both planet and people.

From 1940 to 1960 some two hundred pesticides were created to kill insects, weeds, rodents, and other organisms considered to be "pests."

The first man-made pesticide was DDT, introduced to control malaria and typhus during World War II. DDT was so effective that it was made available to farmers in 1945. In 1973, DDT was banned due to its toxic effects to human health and the environment.

In 1962, Rachel Carson wrote of these pesticides:

> They have entered and lodged in the bodies of fish, birds, reptiles and domestic and wild animals so universally that scientists carrying on animal experiments find it almost impossible to locate subjects free from such contamination. They have been found in fish in remote mountain lakes, in earthworms burrowing in soil, in the eggs of birds—and in man himself. For these chemicals are now stored in the bodies of the vast majority of human beings, regardless of age. They occur in the mother's milk, and probably in the tissues of the unborn child. . . . This situation also means that today the average individual almost certainly starts life with the first deposit of a growing load of chemicals his body will be required to carry henceforth.

Silent Spring beautifully describes the many ways toxic chemicals were, and still are, destroying life—from contaminating surface waters and underground seas, poisoning the soil, disturbing plant communities, silencing songbirds, tainting fish, polluting air, and fouling our food supply to sickening humans, disrupting fertility, and causing cancer. A grassroots uprising followed the publication of her book, and our modern-day environmental movement was born to protect the environment from toxics. Yet still, almost fifty years later, there are more and more toxic chemicals, and damage to our health and the environment continues.

At the time *Silent Spring* was written, toxic pesticides were already widespread in the environment and in the bodies of every living organism, from humans in urban areas to Antarctic penguins. My body, and your body.

And many millions of tons more toxic chemicals of all kinds have been added to our environment since.

In this chapter, you'll learn:

* how toxic chemicals harm the environment
* how toxic chemicals in the environment can damage your health and what you can do
* how you contribute to toxic pollution in the environment and what you can do to reduce your toxic impact
* how you can take action to reduce toxic exposures in your community

The dangers are known. It's now up to each of us to choose to be toxic-free.

How Toxic Chemicals Harm the Environment

Beyond the issue of human toxicity is the question of whether a substance is *ecotoxic*—that is, toxic to other species in the environment and to the sustainability of the functions of the earth.

Ecotoxicity involves the identification of chemical hazards to the environment. According to the EPA, "Ecotoxicity studies measure the effects of chemicals on fish, wildlife, plants, and other wild organisms."

Chemical and pesticide manufacturers submit ecotoxicity studies to regulatory authorities to support the registration and/or approval of their products. Testing on animals or plants to determine whether environmental samples such as soil, sediment, and effluents contain toxic compounds is also called ecotoxicity testing.

Every living thing has its own tolerance for toxics, and the potential for harm to other species is sometimes greater and sometimes less for us. We are much more sensitive to radiation, for example, than are most plants and animals, yet some pesticides are more dangerous to beneficial insects and fish than to humans.

One example of ecotoxicity I experienced in my own life happened in the 1980s when I was living in northern California. The pesticide malathion was sprayed from helicopters over many residential areas to kill the Mediterranean fruit fly. The spraying showed no immediate human health effects, but later the deaths of thousands of fish and the loss of many beneficial insects were linked to the chemical.

The ecotoxicity of a substance is generally determined by evaluating:

- the inherent toxicity of the substance
- its persistence in the environment (biodegradability)
- its tendency to bioaccumulate up the food chain

INHERENT TOXICITY

Establishing the inherent toxicity of a substance is difficult enough in the human species, as sex, age, and health of each individual human body affects how toxic a substance might be in that body.

Imagine, then, how difficult it might be to establish the inherent toxicity of a chemical to millions of different species receiving the exposure—a flower, tree, insect, fish, bird, whale, or any of the other millions of organisms on this earth.

Much is known about toxic exposures to experimental laboratory animals, but beyond that, our knowledge is limited to the toxic effects of only a few chemicals on only a few species of birds and fish. With millions of chemicals and millions of species, that's a lot we do not know about how chemicals are affecting the environment. It is very likely we will never know the toxicity of every chemical to every species, nor all the possible synergistic effects.

Just as an example of how products of varying toxicity can affect an environment, here are some of the results of a study done by the California Department of Fish and Game (Region 3) back in the 1990s on the toxicity of common consumer products that end up in our waterways. They did a test called the LC50 (lethal concentration 50), which shows the concentration in water of any substance that would kill half the aquatic organisms in ninety-six hours (this is actually a theoretical number: they find the concentration at which all die and at which none die, then calculate the concentration at which half die).

PRODUCT	LC50	
Household Bleach	4 ppm	(most toxic)
Natural Solvent Cleaners and Degreasers	31 ppm	
Nokomis All-Purpose Cleaner Concentrate	36 ppm	
All Laundry Detergents	44 ppm	
Sunlight Dish Detergent	49 ppm	
Eagle One Car Wash and Wax, Super Concentrate	114 ppm	
Kelly Moore Premium Acry-Shield Paint	275 ppm	
Amway LOC (Liquid Organic Cleaner)	315 ppm	
Fabergé Organic Shampoo	1,300 ppm	
Kelly Moore Latex Flat Wall Paint	1,650 ppm	
Hydrogen Peroxide (3% solution)	1,675 ppm	
Tone Bar Soap	10,000 ppm	
Hawaiian Punch Fruit Drink	27,500 ppm	(least toxic)

OF COURSE, this data is almost twenty years old and does not necessarily represent the environmental effects of these particular brand-name products today, but it makes the point that the products we use at home *do* end up in the environment and have effects.

I find it interesting that laundry detergents were more toxic to fish than paint(!), even though to humans it is the other way around. But I'm not surprised that household bleach was the most toxic thing they tested, since this is the same hypochlorite used to kill bacteria in our municipal water supplies. Bacteria is bacteria, and chlorine kills bacteria, whether in tap water, a natural waterway, or the intestines of your body.

Throughout this book, I say over and over that the determining factor as to whether or not toxic exposures cause harm to you depends on (1) the toxicity of the poison, and (2) the ability of your body to excrete the poison. This also applies to the planet. Right now, the amount of toxic poisons we humans release into the environment is greater than the amount the planet can handle.

PERSISTENCE IN THE ENVIRONMENT

In our human bodies, there are things we can do to eliminate toxic chemicals. With the earth, however, there is no place for toxic chemicals to be eliminated to.

The earth depends on a cycle of breaking down life forms and recycling molecules into making new life forms, such as a tree making leaves, which fall and return to the soil, where they biodegrade into nutrients that the tree then uses to make new leaves.

Toxic synthetic chemicals with molecular structures that do not break down under normal conditions in the environment violate this law of nature and have a tendency to persist in the environment.

One very visible example of persistence in the environment is the Great Pacific Garbage Patch, a "trash vortex" that stretches from Hawaii to Japan. In this area that is twice the size of the continental United States, more than one hundred million tons of persistent plastic trash has accumulated. Plastic debris in this area causes the deaths of more than a million seabirds every year, and more than one hundred thousand marine mammals. Syringes, cigarette lighters, and toothbrushes have been found inside the stomachs of dead seabirds that mistook them for food. While these accumulated plastics are not directly toxic to us, they demonstrate quite dramatically how man-made chemicals do persist in the environment.

Another example of a persistent man-made chemical that is not so visible but is much more toxic is **polychlorinated biphenyl (PCB)**. PCBs are oil additives that were developed soon after the use of electricity became widespread, because electrical equipment needed oil that didn't break down. Now we find that PCBs are toxic and we cannot escape them because they persist in the environment.

This is true for most other man-made substances as well, unless they are specifically designed to biodegrade.

BIOACCUMULATION

Bioaccumulation occurs when an organism absorbs a toxic substance at a rate greater than that at which the substance is lost. It's like a bathtub. If you are running water into a bathtub faster than it can flow out through the drain, water will accumulate in the bathtub. The same principle applies to every plant and animal, and to the planet as a whole.

Bioaccumulation then multiplies up through the food chain. Persistent substances that are not easily broken down accumulate in organisms low on the food chain, which in turn are eaten by predators higher up. As you go up the food chain, each higher predator has a greater and greater accumulation.

Humans, at the top of the food chain, are one of the most bioaccumulative organisms on the planet, because we take in all the poison pollutants bioaccumulated at every level of the food chain. The result is that we all carry around high levels of chemicals in our fat that in the environment are at much lower levels, and pass this accumulation on to our offspring.

Bioaccumulation makes it very difficult to determine ecotoxicity with any kind of accuracy. Even with all the money that might be spent on future environmental tests, we may still never be able to determine ecotoxicity accurately because substances can bioaccumulate in one organism with no visible effects yet be fatally toxic to its predator, and chemicals can subtly interfere with plant and animal behavior or reduce the population of a species affecting the whole predator-prey relationship of an ecosystem.

Obviously we could initiate complex programs that include multi-species tests, ecological testing preserves, and mathematical ecosystem models to give us accurate data. But is the effort worth it? Perhaps the health and environmental costs of using toxic man-made chemicals have already exceeded their benefits.

As your body ages, it accumulates more and more toxic chemicals.

The same holds true for other species and the planet as a whole. The more toxic waste we dump into the environment, the more polluted the planet becomes. And then *we breathe that polluted air, drink that polluted water, and eat food grown in that polluted soil.*

EVALUATING THE ECOTOXICITY OF CONSUMER PRODUCTS

Unfortunately, at present we, as consumers, cannot completely evaluate ecotoxicity on a product-by-product basis because we don't have adequate information on the toxics released into the environment during manufacture, use, or disposal. And there is little research available on the ecotoxicity of various chemicals.

For now, the best we can do for most substances is assume that if it is toxic to humans, it is probably also toxic to the environment, and that if a product contains a known toxic substance, its manufacture probably produces toxic waste.

You can find limited data on the environmental effects of chemicals in Section 12 of a material safety data sheet for a product or chemical (see Appendix E: How to Read a Material Safety Data Sheet [MSDS]).

How Toxics in the Environment Can Damage Your Health, and What You Can Do to Protect Yourself

There are many ways you might encounter toxic chemicals as you travel through your community on a given day.

The first step to doing something to reduce your exposure is to become aware of what toxic chemicals you might be exposed to, what their health effects are, and where you might be exposed to them. Then you can make a plan to minimize your risk and explore how you can help to reduce the presence of these toxic substances in your community, so everyone can be safe and healthy and all life in the environment can thrive too.

TOXIC CHEMICALS IN YOUR COMMUNITY

Just as there are toxic chemicals in the environment of your home, there are also toxic chemicals in the environment of the community where you live.

These chemicals can pollute the air, water, and soil. They come from sources such as:

- factories
- construction sites
- transportation exhausts (cars, buses, trucks, trains, airplanes)
- brownfields (properties that were once used for commercial or industrial purposes, are now targeted for redevelopment, and are where hazardous substances may be present; examples of brownfields include abandoned factories, gas stations, oil storage facilities, and other businesses that used polluting substances)
- farms
- landfills
- schools
- parks
- homes
- office buildings and stores
- commercial and recreational ship exhaust near ports

There is a great website called Tox Town: Environmental Health Concerns and Toxic Chemicals Where You Live, Work, and Play (www .toxtown.nlm.nih.gov) that gives a comprehensive overview of the toxic chemicals you might encounter—and their health effects—in the type of environment where you live or are visiting: city, town, farm, U.S.-Mexico border, and port.

Another helpful site is MyEnvironment, run by the EPA (www.epa .gov/myenvironment). Here you can enter a location (your address, a zip code, a park name, etc.) and get air quality information, public health data, toxic releases for the area, superfund sites, brownfields, hazardous wastes, water conditions, watershed data, and much, much more.

And there is also the Right-to-Know Network (www.rtknet.org), which gives access to government-held information on the environment, health, and safety. Here you can find information on toxic releases, spills and accidents, risk management, hazardous waste, and more.

All three of these sites will lead you to other sites that have data about toxic exposures where you live.

Outdoor Air Pollution

Though studies show that indoor air pollution is generally greater than outdoor air pollution (if you are using toxic products in your home), outdoor air pollution can be pretty toxic, too, depending on where you live. To find out how polluted the air is where you live, visit the American Lung Association's State of the Air website (www.stateoftheair.org).

Your respiratory system is designed to protect your lungs from germs and large particles like dust and pollen. However, toxic chemicals in air pollution bypasses those defenses, causing harm to them and to lung tissue. Air pollution can make your eyes water, irritate your nose, mouth, and throat, and make you cough and wheeze. But the most common air pollutants can also cause more dangerous health effects, including:

* premature death
* shortness of breath and chest pain
* increased risk of asthma attacks
* chronic obstructive pulmonary disease (COPD), a group of diseases, including emphysema and chronic bronchitis, that share the common symptom of breathlessness

In addition, once inhaled, air pollutants can be absorbed into your bloodstream and reach all areas of your body.

Next time you check your local weather forecast, listen for the air quality index (AQI) report. This system exists to warn the public when air pollution is dangerous. It tracks ozone (smog) and particle pollution (tiny particles from ash, vehicle exhaust, soil dust, pollen, and other pollution). Newspapers and radio and television stations report AQI levels year-round or you can go to the www.airnow.gov website for information.

What you can do to protect yourself:
- When unhealthy levels of air pollution occur, stay indoors as much as possible.
- If you have many days with unhealthy air, consider getting an air filter (see page 39).
- Avoid exercising near high-traffic areas.
- Walk or bike on side streets with less traffic.

Water

Water is continuously moving through our bodies and the environment in an immense cycle. It falls to the ground as rain or snow, then runs into lakes and rivers (surface water) or percolates into the ground (groundwater). It eventually flows to the oceans and evaporates into the sky, where it forms into clouds, and the cycle starts all over again. And when rain falls through the sky, it collects air pollutants along the way.

We humans interrupt this cycle by taking water from surface or underground sources (via wells) for our own use, and then put wastewater back into the cycle.

Toxic contaminants in source water range from arsenic and cadmium from fossil fuel combustion to pesticide runoff from agriculture and industrial-waste leaks.

The most recent contamination of concern has been the discovery of pharmaceutical residues in various water sources. Drugs such as antibiotics, antidepressants, birth control pills, seizure medication, cancer treatments, painkillers, tranquilizers, and cholesterol-lowering compounds have been found, many of which come from household toilets. These drugs can pass intact through conventional sewage treatment facilities and into waterways, lakes, and even aquifers. Discarded pharmaceuticals often end up at dumps and landfills, where they can enter underlying groundwater.

Residues from personal-care products are also showing up in water. Usually these chemicals are the active ingredients or preservatives in cosmetics, toiletries, or fragrances. Some are known to be persistent toxic chemicals. Some sunscreen agents have been detected in lakes and fish as well.

What you can do to protect yourself:
- Find out what is in your water that you need to protect yourself from. Get your water tested.
- Buy a water filter that will sufficiently remove the pollutants that are in your water. At the moment, current water filters do not remove pharmaceuticals.
- Drink bottled water from a reliable source, bottled in glass.

Soil and Food

Many pollutants from the air fall to the ground and enter the soil. Here they may be transformed into harmless nutrients or chemicals even more toxic than the original substance.

Eventually all soil pollutants meet one of four fates:

- They may be taken up by plants growing in the soil, and then eaten by humans or by other animals that are then eaten by humans.
- They may be flushed out of the soil by rainwater into bodies of water, where they become water pollutants (pesticides applied to food and fiber crops often meet this fate).
- If the pollutant is sufficiently volatile, it could rise into the atmosphere and become an air pollutant, where it can then travel great distances.
- Some toxic metals simply stay in the soil forever because they are not volatile, or soluble in water, and cannot be taken up by plants.

What you can do to protect yourself:
Eat organically grown food. But keep in mind that even organically grown food may contain residues of toxics that are present in the soil. At least, there are no added toxics in organically grown food.

How You Contribute to Toxic Pollution in the Environment, and What You Can Do to Reduce Your Toxic Impact

Things we do at home can cause pollution in the environment, which we are then exposed to through air, water, and food. But when we clean up the environment to safeguard our own health, all other species and ecosystems benefit too.

Here are five ways you may be contributing to toxic environmental pollution in your everyday life—and some things you can do to reduce your impact.

HOME ENERGY USE

When you turn on a light, or plug in an electric appliance, do you think about the toxic chemicals you are releasing into the environment?

Even though electricity is toxic-free in your home, it's not toxic-free in the environment. Here is where our electricity comes from in the United States:

- 49.8 percent from burning coal
- 19.9 percent from nuclear power
- 17.9 percent from natural gas
- 6.5 percent from hydroelectric facilities
- 3 percent from burning petroleum
- 2.3 percent from renewable energy sources such as wind power, solar energy, geothermal power, and biomass (plant material used as fuel)

That's 97.7 percent of our electricity putting toxic emissions and greenhouse gases into the air every time we use a kilowatt.

Reduce Your Toxic Impact

Use less energy in your home. By reducing energy use, you can help improve air quality, curb greenhouse gas emissions, encourage energy independence, and save money! Some things you can do:

- Change your lightbulbs to bulbs that use less energy, such as halogens (not compact fluorescents or LEDs because they contain toxic substances—see page 105).
- Choose Energy Star qualified products in more than fifty categories (www.energystar.gov).
- Save on heating and cooling by changing air filters regularly and getting your HVAC tuned annually.
- Use water efficiently. Municipal water systems use a lot of energy to purify and distribute water to households. Saving water, especially hot water, can reduce air pollution.
- Buy recycled products. Products made from recycled materials use less energy in the manufacturing process than virgin materials, creating less air pollution. Better yet, buy or swap for "gently used" products that can be given a second life with you before they are discarded. Check out garage sales, swap meets, secondhand stores, antique stores, and other places that sell secondhand goods, which require no additional energy at all.
- Use renewable energy, such as solar or wind power. If you can't afford to generate this electricity yourself, purchase renewable energy certificates (aka green tags, green energy certificates, and tradable renewable certificates). These were created by the EPA to make it easy for homeowners to participate in using renewable energy. Each certificate represents the delivery of a specific amount of renewable power (usually one megawatt-hour) into a regional or national energy "grid." This displaces the nonrenewable fossil fuels that would have otherwise been used with nonpolluting energy from solar, wind, biomass, and other renewable sources. When you buy green energy certificates equivalent to the amount of energy you use in your home, you can completely offset the environmental effects of your own energy use, because someone, somewhere along the grid, is using the renewable energy paid for by your certificate.

CAR EXHAUST

When you drive a car, you contribute to the number one source of air pollution. Exhaust fumes cause air pollution, cancer, lead poisoning, and a variety of bronchial and respiratory illnesses.

The average car emits more than one thousand pollutants, including **carbon monoxide**, **nitrogen dioxide**, **sulfur dioxide**, **benzene**, **formaldehyde**, **aluminum**, **lead**, **cadmium**, **arsenic**, and **harmful particles**.

Most cars use gasoline or diesel for fuel. These are derived from crude oil. And obtaining oil involves oil spills. Living here on the Gulf Coast of Florida, I was horrified in 2010 at the environmental and health effects of the Gulf Coast spill, which continue today.

Reduce Your Toxic Impact

- Buy local. Every product you buy that is shipped from another place carries within it "embodied" pollution from shipping. Make things yourself from locally available materials; seek out local artisans and craftspeople; support local businesses.
- Reduce the amount of exhaust you produce by carpooling and combining trips. You will also save money on fuel.
- Use public transportation, particularly if your local public transportation uses clean fuels (if they don't, encourage them to do so). Use buses, subways, light-rail systems, commuter trains, or other alternatives to driving your car.
- Use hand-powered or electric lawn care equipment rather than gasoline-powered. Two-stroke engines like lawn mowers and leaf and snow blowers often have no pollution control devices. They can pollute the air even more than cars. Better yet, turn your lawn into an organic vegetable garden and recycle the metals in your lawn mower.
- Consider alternative fuels. A friend of mine has two vehicles he runs on vegetable oil, an old Mercedes-Benz and a pickup truck. Yes, straight vegetable oil. The exhaust emissions from vegetable oil are far less toxic, and the vegetable oil is in your kitchen cupboard!
- Check out the World Carfree Network (www.worldcarfree.net) for ideas on how we can create a car-free society.

PESTICIDES

Pesticides are involved with many household activities. In addition to the obvious pesticides used around your home and garden to kill insects, pesticides are also on your food and used to grow natural fibers, particularly cotton.

Pesticides as a group are particularly toxic to many species, including humans, and tend to persist in the environment. It's best to just not use them in the first place.

Reduce Your Toxic Impact

- Buy organically grown food that is grown and raised without pesticides.
- Buy organically grown natural fibers. Cotton in particular uses a lot of pesticides in the growing of crops. Though cotton fabric is toxic-free to our health by the time it goes through processing from fiber to fabric, it's not toxic-free to the environment.
- Learn to control pests around your home without pesticides (see page 60).
- Learn organic gardening methods so you don't need pesticides in your garden.

TOXIC HOUSEHOLD PRODUCTS

Whenever you use household products known to be toxic, there is likely to be toxic waste put into the environment. In 2007 (the most recent year for which data was available), the United States put 34.7 million tons of hazardous waste into the environment. That's 69.5 billion pounds of toxic waste released into our air, water, and soil.

Four types of industry account for about 90 percent of industrial hazardous wastes generated in the United States: chemical manufacturing, primary metal production, metal fabrication, and petroleum processing.

And all of these industries are making consumer products you are using every day.

Reduce Your Toxic Impact

- Buy toxic-free products that do not produce toxic waste in their manufacture or disposal (see Chapter 2: Home).

GLOBAL SHIPPING POLLUTION

Whenever you purchase a product made in another country, you contribute to air pollution from global shipping.

The American Lung Association, the Environment Defense Fund, and other groups are working to establish an emissions control area in U.S. waters to protect the health of Americans from global shipping pollution.

According to their report *Protecting American Health from Global Shipping Pollution*, oceangoing ships impact air quality in U.S. coastal cities and ports and even send pollution hundreds of miles inland.

The health effects of diesel emissions in general are well documented. Diesel air pollution from these ships adds to cancer risk all around the United States. And because diesel emissions contain a complex mixture of chemicals, exposure to shipping pollution contributes to a wide range of other health risks, including pulmonary disease, cardiovascular effects, neurotoxicity, low birth weight in infants, premature births, congenital abnormalities, and elevated infant mortality rates.

Particulate matter in shipping exhaust can aggravate respiratory conditions such as asthma and chronic bronchitis and has been associated with heartbeat irregularities, heart attacks, and premature deaths.

Reduce Your Toxic Impact

- Buy toxic-free products made in the United States.

Community Action

Because much of our exposure to toxics happens on a community level, we need to begin to address toxics exposure as a public health issue.

We need to help each other learn about toxic exposures and toxic-free alternatives, as well as stand together to clean up existing toxics and prevent new toxic exposures from coming into our community.

Every community is unique and has its own toxic exposures to clean up, from pesticides used in public parks to toxic-waste dumping.

Take a look around and see if there is a group working to clean up toxics in your community. If not, organize one.

The Center for Health, Environment & Justice (www.chej.org) was founded by Lois Gibbs in 1981 after winning the nation's first community relocation of nine hundred families due to a leaking toxic-waste dump in Love Canal, New York. They have many resources available for taking community action regarding toxics and can help you with specific toxic exposures in your community. In particular, see their BE SAFE Campaign for Precautionary Action.

Also see the Women's Health & the Environment (www.womens healthandenvironment.org) "In Your Community" section for more ideas on how you can clean up toxics in your community.

CHAPTER 4

Body

We now know that everybody in America—and around the world—carries toxic chemicals inside their bodies every moment of every day. . . . Everyone has a problem and everyone needs a solution.

—JOHN PETERSON MYERS
coauthor, *Our Stolen Future* (1996)

ONCE YOU have reduced your exposure to toxic chemicals coming *into* your body, the next step toward health is to take chemicals *out* of your body.

Of course, taking chemicals out of your body is always helpful even if you don't eliminate your toxic exposures, but to detox your body without detoxing your home is like trying to empty a bathtub while at the same time having the faucet open, refilling the tub with water.

If you truly want good health, you need to do both.

For almost three decades I had enough success improving my

health by eliminating exposures to toxic chemicals in my home that I thought all I needed to do was live in a nontoxic home and my body would heal itself because it wasn't being bombarded with toxic chemicals. This was true . . . to a degree I thought I was satisfied with.

And then one day my nutritionist gave me a little bottle of tasteless, odorless detox drops that made my body feel so much better so fast, it was like a new awakening for me. It was life-changing.

Before, all I could do was avoid toxic chemicals. Now I could do something to make my body more able to withstand the toxic chemicals I couldn't avoid.

The change was so dramatic, I had to admit that simply avoiding toxic chemicals in my home wasn't enough to get my body to the level of health I wanted.

After taking the drops for ten days, I made a list of all the ways my body had improved since starting to take them. Here's what I wrote:

Improvement Remarkable
- sleeping better
- when I wake up, body is refreshed
- have good energy, but not hyper
- clear mind
- feeling happy and cheerful
- feeling like I have the energy to do whatever I want
- digestive tract improvement
- suddenly scheduling evening social activities instead of resting
- getting a lot of work done
- not feeling stressed
- don't feel like I'm "slogging through the mud"
- eyesight noticeably better
- wanting to go for a walk instead of making myself exercise

After three weeks on these detox drops, I went to the dentist to get my teeth cleaned. The hygienist said, "What are you doing? This is by far the best checkup you've ever had." The condition of my gums had noticeably improved. I told her I had been taking detox drops and she said they absolutely could be helping, because as you detox your body, everything in your mouth improves.

After four weeks my nutritionist said, "Wow! Your body is so strong today! Are you lifting weights or something?" I said no, not a bit of exercise of any kind. But my body did feel unusually strong and I could feel muscles forming as if I had been lifting weights.

People started to notice that I looked different—more alive and vibrant. One day a woman thought I even sounded better over the phone! Everyone wanted to know what I was doing.

As I continued to take the detox drops, my overall health just continued to improve and improve. Most noticeable was that I could work long hours during the day and still have energy to go to meetings or socialize in the evenings. My blood sugar improved. I was just happier, too, getting out from under the depressive effects of toxic substances in my body.

Seeing my improvement, a man I know decided to take these detox drops as well, and the change in him was . . . well, he was like a new man. After he had been taking the drops for about a month, I could see a huge difference in him. Prior to taking the drops, he could only work five or six hours a day and then he would need to rest and would be too tired to do anything else. After taking the drops for two weeks, he worked on a construction job where he was doing heavy labor in 95-degree heat, nine to eleven hours a day, every day. Over the weekend too. At age fifty-six. He would just go home and eat and sleep and go back out to work again with no complaints and in a happy mood. And he started feeling more romantic too. . . .

The detox drops I take contain activated liquid zeolite (read more about this on page 170).

I had such a success with these detox drops that I became very interested in the whole subject of detoxing the body. Taking these drops turned out to be just the beginning of detox for me. I decided that if this method of detox worked so well, I should look into how I could support the natural detox system of my body.

In this chapter, you'll learn:

- all about your body's detox system
- how you can support your detox system with simple good health practices
- how you can protect and strengthen your detox organs to restore your body's natural detoxification function
- how you can remove toxic chemicals from your body

While there are many things you can do yourself to aid your body in processing and removing toxic chemicals, you may also wish to get some professional help. In fact, if you really want to thoroughly detox your body, get professional help. Professionals have products and techniques available that are not accessible to the general consumer. Some of these are more powerful and effective and thus require supervision. But also, professionals have more knowledge and experience and can guide you through the experience successfully.

If you want professional assistance handling the effects of toxic exposures, look for:

- **a naturopathic doctor**
  Naturopathic doctors use diet, exercise, lifestyle changes, and cutting-edge natural therapies along with modern medical science to restore health. (American Association of Naturopathic Physicians [www.naturopathic.org])
- **a doctor who practices environmental medicine**
  Doctors who practice environmental medicine are medical professionals who treat illnesses that are related to toxic chemical exposures. (American Academy of Environmental Medicine [www.aaemonline.org]; Association of Occupational and Environmental Clinics [www.aoec.org])
- **a doctor who practices functional medicine**
  Doctors who practice functional medicine deal with primary prevention and underlying causes of illness instead of symptoms. They examine core clinical imbalances that underlie various disease

conditions, which arise as environmental inputs such as diet, nutrients (including air and water), exercise, and traumas are processed by one's body, mind, and spirit. (Institute for Functional Medicine [www.functionalmedicine.org])

- **a doctor who practices anti-aging medicine**
Anti-aging doctors use advanced scientific and medical technologies for the early detection, prevention, treatment, and reversal of age-related diseases and to prolong the healthy lifespan in humans. (American Academy of Anti-Aging Medicine [www.world health.net])

- **a certified clinical nutritionist**
A Certified Clinical Nutritionist uses nutrition to achieve normal physiological function. (The International & American Associations of Clinical Nutritionists [www.iaacn.org])

- **a chiropractor**
Doctors of chiropractic focus on disorders of the musculoskeletal system and the nervous system, and the effects of these disorders on general health. However, many also offer other complementary natural remedies including nutrition and detoxification. (American Chiropractic Association [www.acatoday.org]; American Chiropractic Council on Nutrition [www.councilonnutrition.com])

- **a biologic dentist**
Biologic dentists work closely with other health care professionals—nutritionists, chiropractors, bodyworkers, naturopaths, and environmental doctors—to reduce the toxic burden to the body as a result of toxic materials used in dental work. (Consumers for Dental Choice [www.toxicteeth.org]; Holistic Dental Association [www .holisticdental.org]; International Academy of Biological Dentistry and Medicine [www.iabdm.org]; International Academy of Oral Medicine and Toxicology [www.iaomt.org]; International Association of Mercury Free Dentists [www.dentalwellness4u.com])

Of course, not all doctors within these specialties will be familiar with toxic chemical exposure and body detoxification, but this is where you will find the doctors and practitioners that are.

Your Body's Detoxification System

To sustain life, your body system needs inputs of food, water, and air and—equally as important—it needs to eliminate wastes. When your body doesn't eliminate wastes, it's like having the garbage in your home pile up because you haven't put it outside in the garbage can to be taken away. Not a very pretty sight either way.

Your body has many ways to eliminate the toxic chemicals that may cause it harm. Every minute of every day, your body is at work draining and purifying itself through the excretion of urine and feces as well as sweat and every breath you exhale.

Your body has five detox organs that make up your "detox system," collectively called the emunctories (from the Latin *emunctus*, past participle of *ex mungere*—"to blow one's nose"):

- liver and intestines (which work together)
- kidneys
- lungs
- skin

If your body is healthy, with good function, toxic chemicals that enter your body are transported to these organs through your blood and your lymph system.

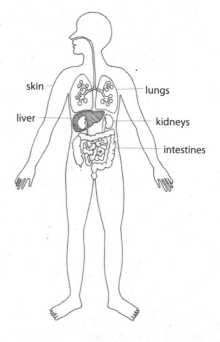

When the primary emunctories fail, your body will continue to try to eliminate toxics through secondary emunctories, which are all the mucous membranes of your body. Many symptoms of illness that we think of as common—such as coughing, sneezing, vomiting, diarrhea, excessive urination, and mucous membrane secretions—are actually your body at work, trying to remove substances that do not belong within it. Keep in mind that these symptoms are the second-line effort after the first emunctories have failed, so if you have these symptoms, they may be indicators that your detox system needs some help. These are also the symptoms that are frequently suppressed with over-the-counter drugs or natural remedies. It's actually better to let your body use these symptoms to remove toxics from your body, rather than try to "relieve" them with a drug or natural remedy.

When the secondary emunctories fail to detox your body, your body will begin to store toxics it cannot excrete. They may accumulate in your joints as arthritis or gout. They may affect your brain and show up as fatigue, depression, or memory loss. When your sweat glands fail to do their job of detoxing your body, your skin tries to drain toxics through its oil glands, resulting in rashes, acne, and eczema.

Just as lack of fiber in food slows defecation and not drinking enough water reduces urination, when liver function is hampered by alcoholic beverages, or when sweat is stopped by an antiperspirant or breathing is diminished by cigarette smoke, or when these systems are compromised in any other way, detoxification becomes less and less efficient, and over time illness occurs.

How toxic chemicals in consumer products and in the environment affect the health of your individual body depends entirely on the condition of your body's detoxification system. So it is very important for you to understand how your body's detox system works and how to keep it in tip-top condition.

How Toxics Move Through Your Body

Because your body needs to eliminate things that don't belong in it, it has natural systems of purification and elimination to keep the whole body system running smoothly.

Toxic chemicals enter your body through:

- injection into the skin (such as drugs)
- ingestion through the mouth (such as pesticides in food)

- absorption through the skin (such as chlorine while taking a shower or swimming in a pool)
- inhalation through the nose (such as vapors of toxic chemicals in cleaning products)

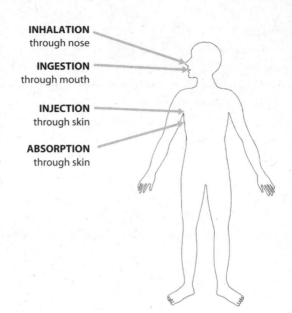

INHALATION
through nose

INGESTION
through mouth

INJECTION
through skin

ABSORPTION
through skin

After a toxicant enters your body, it moves throughout your body:

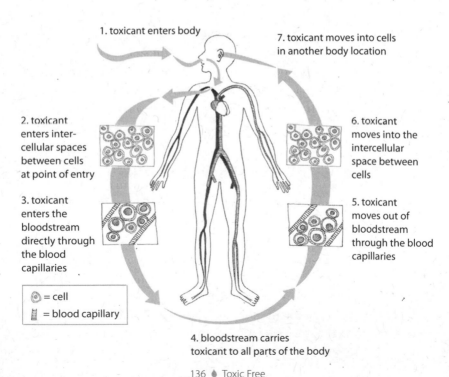

1. toxicant enters body

7. toxicant moves into cells in another body location

2. toxicant enters intercellular spaces between cells at point of entry

6. toxicant moves into the intercellular space between cells

3. toxicant enters the bloodstream directly through the blood capillaries

5. toxicant moves out of bloodstream through the blood capillaries

◎ = cell
▤ = blood capillary

4. bloodstream carries toxicant to all parts of the body

YOUR BLOOD will transfer toxic chemicals into your cells until the amount of that chemical in a cell is equal to the amount of that chemical in your blood. So the more toxicant you have in your blood, the more will go into your cells.

Your body can minimize the potential damage of absorbed toxicants by excreting the chemical:

- through your kidneys as urine
- through your liver via bile, which goes into your intestines and leaves your body through the stool
- through your skin via sweat
- through your lungs as you exhale

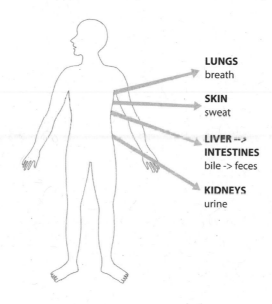

LUNGS
breath

SKIN
sweat

LIVER -->
INTESTINES
bile -> feces

KIDNEYS
urine

YOUR KIDNEYS

The most common pathway through which toxicants are excreted from your body is through your kidneys. Only water-soluble toxicants are excreted through your kidneys (fat-soluble chemicals that come through the kidneys are routed back to be reabsorbed by your body).

The function is very simple:

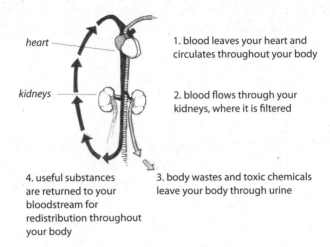

heart — 1. blood leaves your heart and circulates throughout your body

kidneys — 2. blood flows through your kidneys, where it is filtered

4. useful substances are returned to your bloodstream for redistribution throughout your body

3. body wastes and toxic chemicals leave your body through urine

YOUR LYMPHATIC SYSTEM, a part of your immune system, also collects excess, unnecessary, and dangerous materials from cells throughout your body and eliminates them through your kidneys as urine.

Lymph (from the Latin *lympha*, which means "water") is a clear fluid that originates as plasma, the fluid portion of blood, and then turns back into plasma.

Unlike the circulatory system, which moves blood through your body as a result of being pumped by your heart, your lymphatic system does not have a pump to aid its flow. *In order for your lymph system to flow, you must move your body.* This is why exercise is so important for detoxification.

Some toxic chemicals go into the interstitial fluid between the cells, where they are then carried into the cells along with the nutrients, oxygen, and hormones. So, keeping the lymph moving is a very important part of moving chemicals that come into your body out of your body.

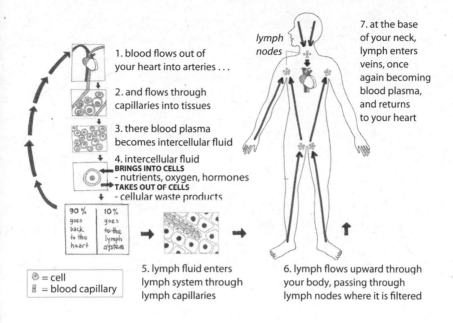

1. blood flows out of your heart into arteries ...

2. and flows through capillaries into tissues

3. there blood plasma becomes intercellular fluid

4. intercellular fluid
BRINGS INTO CELLS
- nutrients, oxygen, hormones
TAKES OUT OF CELLS
- cellular waste products

90% goes back to the heart

10% goes to the lymph system

= cell
= blood capillary

5. lymph fluid enters lymph system through lymph capillaries

6. lymph flows upward through your body, passing through lymph nodes where it is filtered

lymph nodes

7. at the base of your neck, lymph enters veins, once again becoming blood plasma, and returns to your heart

YOUR LIVER AND INTESTINES

Your liver is the second major route for the elimination of toxicants from your body. Here is the process:

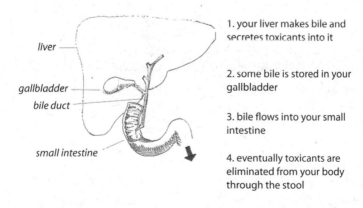

liver

gallbladder

bile duct

small intestine

1. your liver makes bile and secretes toxicants into it

2. some bile is stored in your gallbladder

3. bile flows into your small intestine

4. eventually toxicants are eliminated from your body through the stool

YOUR LIVER processes fat-soluble toxicants into a water-soluble state so your body can excrete them. Why must fat-soluble toxicants be converted to water soluble? If toxicants remain fat-soluble, they would easily dissolve into your fat tissues and fat cells and be stored there for a long time.

Your body prevents long-term storage of fat-soluble chemicals by converting them into water-soluble chemicals in your liver. Then these water-soluble chemicals can be removed from your body via urine or bile.

Excretion of a toxicant through the bile does not necessarily result in the elimination of the toxicant from the body, however. Bile containing the toxicant is dumped into the small intestine, and the chemical must then travel all through the small and large intestines before it leaves the body. If progress is slow through the intestines, or your intestines are not functioning well, there are many opportunities for toxicants in the bile to be reabsorbed by the intestine and in turn reenter the liver. This cycling and recycling of a toxicant can continue indefinitely, keeping the toxicant in the body.

Your liver can make many toxic chemicals harmless, but its ability to do so is greatly affected by:

- the relationship between the size of your liver and the amount of your exposure (a child, for example, has less capacity than an adult)
- the health of your liver
- how much the liver has to work to detoxify your body

Your liver can handle an occasional exposure to toxic chemicals, but frequent exposure stresses your liver and makes it less effective. And we all have frequent exposure to toxic chemicals, to greater or lesser degree.

And if your liver is busy processing toxic chemicals, it has fewer resources available to perform the more than five hundred other functions it is responsible for to maintain the health of your body (see page 197).

YOUR SKIN

Your skin is the home of your sweat glands.

Your body sweats as a natural means of purification. In addition to the critical function of regulating the temperature of your body to 98.6

degrees Fahrenheit, sweat rids your body of poisons and metabolic wastes and helps keep your skin clean, supple, and healthy. Because it eliminates wastes, skin is sometimes called the "third kidney."

The process of sweat is very simple:

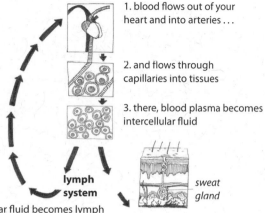

1. blood flows out of your heart and into arteries . . .

2. and flows through capillaries into tissues

3. there, blood plasma becomes intercellular fluid

lymph system

sweat gland

5. some of the intercellular fluid becomes lymph and enters the lymph system, where it is then filtered by your kidneys and returns to your heart

4. some of the intercellular fluid becomes sweat and leaves your body through your sweat glands

⊚ = cell
▌ = blood capillary

WATER-SOLUBLE chemicals and fat soluble chemicals that have been transformed into water-soluble substances are found in sweat.

By itself, sweat is not a major route of excretion of chemicals; however, accelerated by rigorous use of a sauna, it becomes a very effective method for removing toxic chemicals from the body (see page 168).

YOUR LUNGS

Your lungs excrete waste gas molecules from your body, like carbon dioxide, which is made by your body, and gas toxicants from your blood.

Quite simply:

- Tissues in your body lose gas molecules to your blood, which carries them to your lungs to be excreted.
- Specialized cells called alveoli process the molecules captured from the blood into gas and expel the gas when you breathe out.

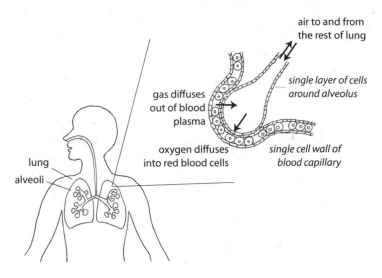

A BREATHALYZER, which measures how much alcohol someone has been drinking, is a good example of how toxic gases can be expelled by the lungs. Even though someone drinks alcohol, it goes throughout the body. The amount of alcohol in a person's breath is a very accurate measure of how much alcohol is in their blood. It is also how we can tell when someone has been eating garlic or smoking cigarettes, because the gases come out of the body through the breath.

How You Can Support Your Detox System

Your detoxification system is the most important system of your body because it determines whether or not your body is sick or well. Failure to detox can result in any and every illness and condition (see Appendix A: How Toxics Affect Your Body Systems).

Each body has its own unique detox system. An exposure that might be disabling or even life-threatening to someone else might cause only a mild irritation for you. Put ten people in a room and give them the same toxic exposure and each one will respond differently because of differences in their detox systems.

Even your own detox system can change from day to day.

In addition to the amount of exposure your body has to toxic chemicals, and any disease or damage that may be compromising your detox organs, several other factors can affect how well your detox system is functioning at any given time:

- **Nutrition.** Poor nutrition reduces the ability of your detox system to function. Detox systems require a wide range of specific nutrients to function, including vitamins, minerals, amino acids, and fatty acids. Many enzymes require a particular vitamin and/or mineral in order to function. If the nutrients are not present, the enzyme becomes paralyzed or inactive, and detoxification cannot take place.
- **Water.** Lack of water slows down detoxification processes.
- **Exercise.** Exercise is necessary for the lymph system to move toxicants out of your body. A sedentary lifestyle slows detoxification processes and leads to a buildup of toxics in your body.

Detoxification is a natural, normal function of your body. Every minute of every day, your body is collecting and removing waste products and foreign matter that does not belong within your system. So it's not about doing an occasional detox "program"; it's about supporting your body's detox system as an ongoing activity, every day.

Since every individual body is different, some methods of detox support will work better than others for you. You may need to try different methods and products to see which one works best for you. Here are the basics.

GET GOOD NUTRITION

Given proper nutrition, the human body has an amazing ability to heal itself. If properly fed and given the right nutrients, the human body is designed to repair and restore all its functions.

Good nutrition can actually protect your body from many toxic exposures. One study found that high doses of vitamin C protected workers from the harmful effects of benzene, a very toxic solvent. Conversely, too much fat in the diet has been found to increase benzene toxicity.

Our detox systems need a lot of nutrients to process toxic chemicals. If our nutrition is too poor, a small exposure to a toxic substance can have a big negative effect.

It's important to eat a whole-food diet to get the nutrients needed to make your detoxification system work. A diet of junk food reduces your detox system's ability to function and detox your body.

Eat Fresh, Local, Organic Foods

On every list I've seen of reasons to eat organic food, the number one reason given is to reduce the toxic load on our bodies and the environment. Organic food also has more nutrition than foods grown and raised with toxic chemicals—and it tastes better.

Organic foods are now widely available at many supermarkets and discount warehouse stores as well as natural-food stores. Visit your local farmers' market or find a Community Supported Agriculture (CSA) program that provides a weekly basket from a local farmer for the freshest produce. And there are also many organic foods available online that can be shipped right to your door.

The most nutritious food is locally sourced and organically grown, direct from the farmer—or, if possible, grow your own.

Prepare Your Foods Yourself at Home

Prepared packaged foods contain many toxic contaminants, from food additives to packaging. When you turn fresh ingredients into delicious meals at home yourself, you have total control over everything that goes into your body.

Food preparation can be fun, fast, and creative, as well as tasty.

Eat Fresh Fruits and Vegetables

Fresh fruits and vegetables cleanse, energize, build, and regenerate your body. They are high in fiber and water, which aid in detoxification.

Fruits and vegetables are best eaten raw or lightly steamed to retain their nutrients and enzymes.

Every day for lunch I eat a pound of raw vegetables in a salad. I weighed it out once to see what a pound of vegetables looked like. It was about three-quarters of my big salad bowl. My salad is mostly greens of different kinds, depending on the season, with green onions, cucumbers, tomatoes, and other vegetables as they become available through the year. All I put on it for dressing is two teaspoons of organic olive oil and a sprinkle of Himalayan salt. I add about 3 ounces of protein and enjoy!

You can also make raw vegetable and fruit smoothies. The sweetness of the fruit covers the flavor of the greens.

Or whiz up some vegetables and add some flavorings to make a cold soup.

Eat Natural Salt

Salt, along with the other electrolytes (potassium, calcium, magnesium), help to transport toxic waste across the extracellular space toward the lymphatic and blood vessels.

The problem with salt is not salt in its natural state but, rather, what most people think of as "table salt": industrialized sodium chloride. Your body doesn't need more sodium chloride. What it does need is sufficient natural salt, with its full spectrum of natural minerals, in order for the process of transport across membranes to occur.

You don't need much, but a pinch of sea salt or Himalayan salt can make a difference in how your body functions. In times past, when salt was "salt of the earth," it was considered so valuable to health that it was used as money.

Eat Enough Good Fat

The amount of fat you eat affects how well your body deals with toxic chemicals.

Sixty to 80 percent of your central nervous system, for example, is made from fatty acids. Fat deficiency makes your nervous system vulnerable to the fat-soluble metals, including cadmium, aluminum, chromium, lead, silver, mercury, and titanium.

The key is to eat sufficient fats, not to go overboard. The general calculation for approximate fat needs is to multiply your body weight in pounds by 12 calories, and multiply this sum by 30 percent to equal total calories of fat per day. So if you weigh 150 pounds, you would need to multiply 1,800 calories by 30 percent to equal 540 calories

One tablespoon of butter equals 101 calories, so you could have 5 tablespoons of butter per day. If you're on a low-fat diet, you're probably not getting enough fat to protect your body from fat-soluble chemicals.

The best fats are from organically grown plants and animals, as fat-soluble chemicals from pesticides concentrate in the fat of plants and animals. I eat primarily organic butter, organic grass-fed cream, organic olive oil, and organic coconut oil.

Eat Enough Protein

The main process by which your body removes fat-soluble toxicants happens in the liver. This process converts fat-soluble chemicals—which would otherwise end up being stored in the body—into water-soluble chemicals that can then be excreted via bile through the intestines.

Your liver needs very specific nutrients in order to process fat-soluble toxicants so they can be removed from your body. And one of these is protein.

At one point in the process, a "carrier" molecule attaches to the toxicant molecule and pulls the toxicant molecule out of the blood, into the liver, through the gallbladder, through the small intestine, and out of the body, much like a tugboat pulls a boat out of a harbor.

Your body has over half a dozen detox molecules that can attach to the toxicant. One is glutathione. Glutathione can grab on to hundreds of types of environmental chemicals and drag them right out of the blood into the liver, then to the gallbladder and into the gut, where they are eliminated in the stool.

For every molecule of chemical that is transformed from fat-soluble to water-soluble, your body loses a molecule of glutathione. So in order for your body to have the continuous ability to detox the toxic chemicals you are exposed to every day, you need to keep replenishing glutathione.

Glutathione is created in the body from three amino acids: glycine, glutamic acid, and cysteine. Amino acids are the structural units that make up proteins.

There are twenty amino acids. Eight are "essential" and the others are "nonessential." The essential amino acids cannot be synthesized by the body, so they must be ingested through food. The nonessential amino acids are made by the body from the essential amino acids. The glycine, glutamic acid, and cysteine needed to make glutathione are all nonessential amino acids, but since nonessential amino acids are made from essential amino acids, it all comes down to having enough protein and all the amino acids in order for your body to have enough gluta- thione to detox.

Animal proteins are called complete proteins because they con- tain all eight essential amino acids. Plant proteins are incomplete because they contain only some of the essential amino acids. If you are a vegetarian or vegan and do not want to eat animal protein in any form, please make sure that you are eating a variety of plant foods that ensure you get all eight essential amino acids.

You don't need to eat excessive protein, but you do need to eat *sufficient* protein.

Your body's protein needs depend on your age, body size, and activity level. The general rule of thumb used by nutritionists to cal- culate the protein need of your body is to multiply your body weight in pounds by 0.37 (or in kilograms by 0.8). So if your body weighs 150 pounds, your protein need is 55 grams of protein per day. You'll need to find out how many grams of protein are in an ounce of the protein sources you regularly eat, as it varies, from less than 6 grams per ounce to about 25 grams per ounce. Steak has 7 grams of protein per ounce, so 55 grams would be about 8 ounces of meat. Of course, you would spread this over three meals, so that would be about 3 ounces per meal.

Do research your protein sources and figure out how much you need to eat at each meal to get sufficient protein. And I would add at least a little more to help your detox system. The Top200Foods.com website (www.top200foods.com) lists protein and amino acid sources of food in descending order (as well as calories, fiber, carbohydrates, fat, vitamins, minerals, antioxidants, sugars, and phytosterols).

The best sources of protein are grass-fed organic animals, seafood from pristine waters, and organically grown legumes and nuts.

Get Sufficient Minerals

Like protein, minerals are essential to the liver detoxification process. Without minerals, the process doesn't happen, and toxic chemicals can be stored in your body.

But in addition, lack of minerals provides the opportunity for toxic metals to attach themselves to vacant mineral binding sites. This is so important that taking minerals can detoxify the body by itself. And your body needs minerals in order to utilize vitamins, so it's very important to make sure you are getting all the minerals your body needs.

Since your body cannot manufacture minerals itself, you have to get minerals from the food you eat. And there are many good food sources

MACRO MINERALS	TRACE MINERALS
Calcium	Cobalt
Chloride	Chloride
Magnesium	Chromium
Phosphorus	Copper
Potassium	Fluoride
Sodium	Iodine
Boron	Iron
	Manganese
	Molybdenum
	Selenium
	Zinc

of minerals. However, today most foods are grown in soils that no longer contain the essential minerals provided by nature and therefore do not contain sufficient minerals for your body to maintain good health.

Some organic farmers supplement their soil with minerals, but don't assume that all organically grown food is mineral-rich.

In nature, there are a variety of minerals that all work together and are present in specific proportions. So what you want to get is a "whole" mineral source that includes the "macro" minerals (those needed in large amounts by your body) and "trace" minerals (those needed in very small amounts).

A good mineral supplement generally comes in liquid form and includes both macro and trace minerals.

Take Organic Whole-Food Supplements

Whole-food supplements are made by concentrating foods for use in supplements. These provide nutrients as they are found in nature, with all the cofactors that help assimilation.

Whole-food supplements include alfalfa- and barley-juice powder, bee pollen, bonemeal, brewer's yeast, chlorophyll, wheatgrass juice or powder, cod-liver oil, desiccated liver, kelp, flaxseed oil, lecithin, fresh-water algae (blue-green algae, chlorella, spirulina), sea vegetables such as kelp, enzymes, wheat-germ oil, and minerals from ancient sea, clay, or vegetation beds.

Today it is easy to find whole-food supplements made from organically grown fruits and vegetables.

Take Probiotics

Probiotics (*probiotic* literally means "for life") are microorganisms, specific bacteria, fungi, and yeasts that are a natural, necessary, component of the digestive tract and an integral part of your immune system.

These microorganisms form a living colony within the lining of your digestive tract and are in a mutually beneficial relationship with your body as a whole. There are actually more bacteria in your intestines than there are cells in your body!

Probiotics work together, assisting your body with digestion, nutrient uptake, and immune defense. They also make B vitamins and vitamin K in your body.

When you are born, your body is inoculated with beneficial bacteria and yeast from your mother's milk. If you were not breast-fed, you may not have had the benefit of probiotics since birth. But even if you did receive your birthright probiotics, they are easily destroyed by toxic chemicals.

Even drinking a simple glass of tap water can destroy the probiotics in your intestines. Tap water contains chlorine or chloramines to kill harmful microorganisms in the water, and most water supplies also contain fluoride, but these chemicals kill *all* microorganisms—both harmful and beneficial—whether in tap water or in your gut.

When the beneficial symbiosis of the digestive lining is disrupted, the disease process begins in small increments, usually starting with symptoms like indigestion, gas, bloating, and heartburn/acid reflux. If an imbalance of the digestive flora persists, a progression of ailments can follow as the immune system becomes compromised.

Remember that *half of the detoxification for the entire body occurs in the gut* as toxicants pass through from the liver, so it's important to keep intestines moving and cleaned out. Also, studies show probiotics support liver function and detoxification.

Given the toxic nature of today's food and water, it would be safe to say that *everybody* needs to replenish "friendly flora" to maintain the health of their digestive tract.

A variety of fermented foods has historically been part of traditional diets to continually restore probiotics in the intestines. Including fermented foods such as yogurt, sour cream, kefir, sauerkraut, kimchi, brine pickles, and other traditional fermented foods in your diet can help to restore probiotics.

Yogurt, however, often contains much more sugar than probiotics, so if you choose to eat yogurt, choose plain yogurt. And today's commercial yogurts are not fermented as long as traditional homemade yogurts, so if you are going to eat yogurt as your source of probiotics, it's better to make it yourself at home.

But you may need to do more than eat fermented foods if your intestinal probiotics really need restoration. If you've ever taken an antibiotic or drink tap water that contains chlorine or chloramines, you probably need to take probiotics. If you have any digestive or immune system problems, probiotics will probably help.

Probiotics are sold in powder form, in capsules filled with powder, or in liquid form. They contain live (but dormant) strains of beneficial bacteria, such as *Lactobacillus acidophilus* (*L. acidophilus*) and *Bifidobacterium bifidum* (*B. bifidum*).

The two major considerations when choosing a probiotic are the variety of strains and the number of living cells.

Select a product that has a mix of *Lactobacillus* and *Bifidobacterium* strains. These are the most common beneficial bacteria, are the safest to take, and have been most researched of all probiotics. These are active in both your small and large intestines. Some products contain *prebiotics*, such as FOS and inulin, which are non-digestible food components that act as "fertilizer" to stimulate the growth of good bacteria.

Read the labels to find out how many organisms are guaranteed to be in each dose. You want at least 1 billion organisms (or cells) per capsule in order for the probiotic to benefit your health.

Take Digestive Enzymes

Digestive enzymes break down food, making nutrients available to be distributed throughout your body. Different enzymes are needed to break down proteins, fats, and carbohydrates.

Your body releases digestive enzymes throughout your digestive tract. The salivary glands in your mouth release the first enzymes that begin to break down food even as you are chewing it. Then, as the food moves to your stomach, more enzymes are released to break down proteins. Still more enzymes are released from your pancreas to break down carbohydrates and fats as the food continues to move through the small intestines.

In addition to making enzymes, your body depends on getting enzymes from the food you eat. If you were an animal living out in the wild (and we do have animal bodies), you would be eating a wide variety of raw plants and animals, all of which contain enzymes.

So why do you need to take a digestive enzyme supplement?

You may not be eating a sufficient amount of the protein and minerals your body needs to make an adequate enzyme supply. And even if you are eating enough nutritious food, your body may not be absorbing the nutrients if your intestines are not in good condition.

And the food you eat may not contain enough enzymes. Enzymes are only available from raw and slightly cooked foods. They are destroyed by heat above 118 degrees. Once enzymes are exposed to heat, they are no longer able to provide the function for which they were designed. Raw foods contain the enzyme "helpers" nature intended for our bodies to have. Cooked food is missing these enzymes and relies on enzymes produced by your body for digestion. And if your body doesn't have enough nutrients to make sufficient enzymes, you need to get some enzymes from somewhere else.

In a natural state, out in the wild, you would eat enzyme-rich foods and your body would produce the enzymes it needed to digest the food you eat. Although it may be theoretically possible to get all your enzymes from food, given the quality of food available today, most people would greatly benefit from taking enzymes.

I myself resisted taking enzymes for a long time, thinking I was getting enough enzymes from the big raw salad I ate almost every day for lunch. But when I started taking an enzyme supplement, I noticed a big difference almost immediately. It was like the food just disappeared once it was in my body. I had more energy and started eating less because I was getting more nutrition from my food. I reduced the amount of supplements I was taking.

One of my very experienced health care providers said to me, "A huge number of people would not need over-the-counter drugs for gastrointestinal problems if they would just take enzymes—even if they don't change their diet at all." The number one thing he does with new clients is have them start taking enzymes.

Another very experienced health care provider said that if I take only one supplement, the one that would do my body the most good is enzymes.

If you need to get some digestive enzymes into your body, eating raw papaya or pineapple with protein will provide enzymes that digest protein, and other raw fruits and vegetables will provide other enzymes. You don't need to go on a 100 percent raw diet; you just need to include some raw food in your diet every day. But I'll just tell you, it's been my experience that this isn't enough.

Because specific enzymes are needed to break down fats, proteins, and carbohydrates, it's best to choose a "broad-spectrum" enzyme product that contains several different enzymes within one product, such as amylase (for carbohydrates), protease (for protein), and lipase (for fats). Enzymes range in price. The stronger ones tend to be more expensive but are well worth the price if your body needs them.

If you have ulcers, choose an enzyme product that does not contain betaine hydrochloride (HCL), as it may irritate your ulcer.

Eat Antioxidants

In your body there is a natural balance of free radicals and antioxidants.

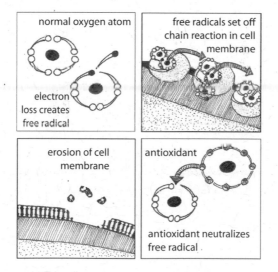

FREE RADICALS (also called reactive oxygen species) are a natural by-product of energy production and other body processes. They are molecules with unpaired electrons on their outer shells. Just like us humans who want to be with a mate, these unpaired electrons are looking to mate up with other electrons. But instead of mating with a "single" electron, they go steal "husbands" and "wives" from other "marriages," destroying those marriages.

To keep free radicals in check, your body has antioxidants. However, exposure to toxic chemicals greatly increases the amount of free radicals in your body, creating an imbalance. With the immense amount of toxic chemicals we all are exposed to, this is the case for most of us.

It is widely known that an excess of free radicals speed the aging process and cause damage to cells or their components. Free-radical damage has been linked to many conditions and diseases, including Alzheimer's, diabetes, cancer, arthritis, and heart disease, as well as premature aging.

The remedy to free radical damage is:

* Reduce the amount of free radicals created by reducing exposure to toxic chemicals and eliminating toxic chemicals from your body.
* Put more antioxidants in your body to restore the balance.

Many foods contain a lot of antioxidants. The antioxidant capacity of foods is expressed in its oxygen radical absorbance capacity (ORAC) value. You can compare the ORAC values of various foods at www .oracvalues.com.

One hundred grams of ground cloves top the list at ORAC 314,446. Acai berries are 102,700 ORAC. Dry cocoa powder is 80,933 ORAC. A lot of herbs and spices have high ORAC values, as do nuts, beans, fruits, and vegetables. Basically, antioxidants are found in plant foods. So if you eat a good, whole-food diet, you'll get lots of antioxidants.

There are many antioxidant products and supplements that have high ORAC values, but my opinion is you can get all the antioxidants you need from food.

If you want to eat chocolate as an antioxidant, here's my recipe for making a quick chocolate treat that doesn't contain toxic sugars or additives.

DEBRA'S CHOCOLATE FUDGE

Makes 1 serving

1 heaping teaspoon organic unsweetened cocoa powder
1 heaping teaspoon your favorite natural sweetener (I use coconut sugar.)
1 teaspoon organic butter, softened
2 teaspoons grass-fed organic cream

Mix all ingredients together in a small bowl and eat it right off the spoon. Start with these measurements and adjust to the consistency you prefer. You can also add flavorings, nuts, and anything else you want to make any flavor chocolate you like. If you put it in the refrigerator, it will firm up and you can roll it into balls for truffles or cut it into squares like fudge.

ORAC 3237

BUT THERE is also another source of free electrons that can neutralize free radicals: the earth.

According to the book *Earthing: The Most Important Health Discovery Ever?* by Clinton Ober, Stephen T. Sinatra, M.D., and Martin Zucker, if your body is connected to the earth, any free radical formed anywhere in your body will be neutralized by electrons flowing into your body from the earth.

In order for this transfer of electrons from earth to body to occur, your body needs to be directly connected to the earth, such as by bare feet on the grass or on a sandy beach. Electrons will pass through natural materials such as leather but not through the industrial plastics and rubber most shoes are made of today. Lie down on the grass or beach in natural fiber clothing for twenty minutes and your whole body will be revitalized with electrons. It's a simple way to combat damage caused by toxic chemicals.

DRINK PLENTY OF WATER

Water makes up about 60 percent of your body weight. Not only is water essential to life, but since it dissolves more substances than any other liquid, water is essential to detoxing your body. It is the key element required to flush wastes from your cells and through your kidneys, including toxic chemicals. Water also improves the movement of food through your intestines, which helps move toxic chemicals out of your body too.

Water can also prevent diseases known to be caused by toxic exposures. A study done at the Center for Human Nutrition at the University of Sheffield, England, found that women who kept their bodies adequately hydrated reduced their risk of breast cancer by 79 percent. Another study, done at the Fred Hutchinson Cancer Research Center in Seattle, showed that women who drink more than five glasses of water a day have a 45 percent reduced risk of colon cancer compared with women who drink less than two glasses of water a day. Perhaps this is because water was reducing buildup of cancer-causing chemicals in the bodies of these women.

Not enough water leads to dehydration, which is the condition of not having enough water in your body to carry out normal functions.

How much water does your body need? The average adult loses about six 8-ounce glasses of water per day through urine and an additional four glasses through breathing, sweating, and bowel movements. Food usually supplies about two glasses of water, thus the common recommendation of eight glasses of water per day to replace the amount of water your body has lost.

The general rule of thumb is to drink half your weight in ounces of water. So if you weigh 150 pounds, that's 75 ounces, divided by 8 ounces equals nine 8-ounce glasses per day. If you weigh 200 pounds you will need about 12½ glasses of water per day.

You may need to increase your total water intake, depending on how much you exercise, the climate you live in, your health condition, and if you're pregnant or breast-feeding.

Don't wait until you are thirsty to drink water, because thirst is an indicator your body is already dehydrated. By the time you feel thirsty, your body has lost more than 1 percent of its water. It's better to drink water regularly throughout the day to replenish vital stores.

In rare cases, too much water can be harmful. Hyponatremia occurs when your body takes in too much water, diluting vital salt levels in the blood. But you would have to greatly exceed the amount of replacement water your body needs for this to occur.

Of course, if you are drinking water with the intent to remove toxic chemicals from your body, you'll want to drink water that does not itself add toxic chemicals to your body. See Bottled Water (page 65) for more information on obtaining toxic-free water.

EXERCISE REGULARLY

Exercise benefits your body in many ways: it can boost your energy level, help you sleep better, improve your mood, keep your weight and blood sugar down, combat chronic diseases, improve your immune system in general, and even perk up your sex life.

But most important, exercise is essential to your body's detoxification process.

Your lymph system bathes every cell in fluid that carries away cellular wastes and toxic chemicals, *but it doesn't move unless your body moves.* Your heart pumps blood through your body, but lymph fluid just sits there until you move your body. The more you move, the more your lymph system carries toxic chemicals out of your cells so they can be routed out of your body.

It doesn't take a lot of exercise, just regular movement. Start out with whatever you can do, and add to it at a comfortable pace.

Walking is great exercise, or bicycling, or swimming, or dancing—whatever you enjoy. My goal is to walk at least a half hour every day. Often I walk an hour, some days not at all, but it all evens out in the end. I love my walks. Sometimes it's nice to have time alone, other times I walk with a friend. Make your exercise time an enjoyable activity, and you will enjoy exercising. Go outside and get fresh air, but stay away from busy streets where there is a lot of toxic car exhaust.

For the purpose of getting your lymph going, it's not about heart rate or sweat, just movement. So even if you are just getting up and down from sitting at your desk or waving your arms while watching television, every movement helps.

The exercise considered to be best for detoxing your body is rebounding on a mini-trampoline, because it is so effective at pumping the lymph fluid through your body.

How You Can Protect and Strengthen Your Detox Organs

In order to detox your body, your detox organs need to be able to function.

Your kidneys need to be able to filter out toxicants, your liver needs to be able to transform fat-soluble toxics into water-soluble substances, your intestines need to be able to carry the toxics from your liver through twenty-five feet of intestine, your skin needs to be able to sweat out toxicants, and your lungs need to be able to breathe to exhale toxic gases.

All your detox organs need to be in optimum condition, but given the amount of toxic chemicals your body has been exposed to, they probably need some help.

Fortunately, there are many things you can do to protect your detox organs from damage and strengthen each individual organ.

This is a very important step, because your body actually won't release the toxic chemicals from storage in fat, bones, and other places until your detox organs are in good enough shape to eliminate them.

Again, because each body is unique, you may need to try different detox support methods and products to find which work best for you.

STRENGTHEN YOUR KIDNEYS

Kidneys are especially delicate because of their high exposure to toxic chemicals in the blood that filters through them. When toxicant and fat deposits accumulate within your kidneys, their function can be impaired.

Odorless and colorless urine is generally an indication that your kidneys are functioning well.

It is especially important for kidney function to drink ten to twelve glasses of water every day. Your kidneys are flushing toxics out of your entire body, so help the process along with lots of water. If you don't drink enough water, your kidneys may become contaminated with metals, causing them to swell, which reduces their ability to efficiently filter toxicants.

Reduce the stress on your kidneys by reducing stimulating foods and drink, such as red meat, foods with refined salt, tea, and coffee. If you are having kidney problems, reduce your intake of all animal proteins.

Increase your intake of foods that strengthen kidney function—fresh fruits and vegetables in general, and in particular:

- quinoa, barley, and millet
- black beans, mung beans, and (of course) kidney beans
- grapes, cranberries, and blueberries
- fennel, onions, spring onions, celery, beets, spinach, string beans, and asparagus
- parsley, chives, garlic, ginger, and cloves
- spirulina

Take an herbal kidney-support product. There are many brands available. For a kidney detox, drink:

- **fresh cranberry juice:** Run a cup of cranberries through the blender with an adequate amount of water and a spoon of freshly squeezed lemon juice.

- **gingerroot tea:** Peel gingerroot and steep several slices in a cup of boiling water to taste.
- **dandelion tea:** Steep as you would any tea.

STRENGTHEN YOUR LIVER

Your liver may be damaged from toxic chemical exposures, drinking alcoholic beverages, or taking certain drugs, making it less able to process toxic substances.

One day I happened to read a story in a women's magazine about how you can lose weight by cleansing your liver. The article was about a three-day liver rejuvenation program developed by Ann Louise Gittleman, Ph.D., author of the best-selling book *The Fat Flush Plan*.

A friend and I tried the three-day program. Both of us noticeably lost weight, and we both felt great. "Cleaner," we both agreed. My friend said it felt like little Pac-Men were running around in his blood, cleaning it out. I felt that too. And so I went and bought and read *The Fat Flush Plan*.

Well, does she have it right! Dr. Gittleman writes, "Not only is the liver the main organ for detoxifying pollutants and chemicals in the body, but this vital organ also is a hidden key to effortless weight loss."

I think the book should be called *The Liver Restoration Plan*. Dr. Gittleman has a whole liver restoration diet that results in weight loss, but it also restores the ability of your liver to detox your body.

Your liver is so important to detoxing your body, I highly recommend you get Dr. Gittleman's book *The Fat Flush Plan*, read it, and follow her advice. But to get you started, here's the three-day plan my husband and I did.

On the first day, you just drink a liver-cleansing "cocktail."

DR. GITTLEMAN'S LIVER CLEANSE "COCKTAIL"

To make enough for one person for one day, place 1 cup all natural, unsweetened cranberry juice and 7 cups pure water in pot. Bring to a boil, then turn off the heat. Place ½ teaspoon cinnamon, ¼ teaspoon ginger, and ¼ teaspoon nutmeg in a tea ball and steep in the liquid for 15 minutes, then discard the spices.

I made this the night before, then chilled it overnight. In the morning, add ¾ cup fresh orange juice and ¼ cup fresh lemon juice.

First thing in the morning, pour 1 cup cleansing cocktail in a glass, add 2 tablespoons ground flaxseed, and drink. An hour later, drink 1 cup water.

For the rest of the day, alternate drinking 1 cup cocktail (without flaxseeds) with drinking 1 cup water. When you get to the last glass of cocktail, add another 2 tablespoons ground flaxseeds and drink.

The next two days, I ate only liver-enhancing foods: eggs, yogurt, artichokes, beets, broccoli and cauliflower, cinnamon, and nutmeg. I didn't eat all of these, I just chose the ones I liked.

CRUCIFEROUS VEGETABLES (of the genus *Brassica*) are highly recommended for liver detox. At least one serving a day is suggested, but even one serving a week can be beneficial. These are the brassicas:

arugula	mustard greens
broccoli	kohlrabi
Brussels sprouts	radishes
cabbage	rutabagas
cauliflower	turnips
collard greens	watercress
kale	

While drinking the cocktail and including liver support foods in my diet did improve the health of my body somewhat and is a good way to start, a few years later I got professional help and did a high-powered, supervised liver detox for two months. I highly recommend professional help with this.

Because the detox pathway for removing toxic chemicals through the liver includes sending chemicals through the intestines to be excreted, supporting liver function also requires supporting intestinal function.

STRENGTHEN YOUR INTESTINES

Intestines carry toxicants from your liver out of your body, so it's important to keep things moving. Toxicants that sit in constipated intestines can be reabsorbed into your body through the intestinal wall.

In addition to drinking sufficient water, and taking probiotics and enzymes, the next most important thing to do is to include at least 35 grams of fiber per day from vegetables and fruits in your diet. You can find a list of high-fiber foods at www.top200foods.com. Some of the top fiber-rich foods are lentils, peas, beans, whole grains, and nuts, followed by fruits and vegetables.

Generally, if you are drinking enough water and eating enough fiber—especially vegetables and fruits—the peristaltic action of your intestines should move food wastes through just fine. If your intestines need a little help, try taking aloe, vitamin C, magnesium, or one of the herbal laxatives available at natural-food stores. But do everything you can to keep your intestines moving by means of a correct diet, as it is unhealthy to become dependent on laxatives.

STRENGTHEN YOUR SKIN

The best way to support your skin as a detox organ is to sweat, as that cleanses your skin from the inside out. Antiperspirants, temperature-controlled indoor environments, synthetic clothing, and physical idleness all conspire to inhibit the healthy flow of sweat. Exercise, sauna or steam baths, and soaking in warm baths all contribute to producing sweat and rejuvenate the skin.

Caring for your skin in certain ways will also get your lymph system moving. One way to stimulate lymph is to brush your whole body every few days with a dry loofah or rough bath brush. This removes flakes of dried skin cells that accumulate on the outer layer of your skin, which can clog the sweat pores through which toxicants are released. Lymphatic massage from a qualified professional will also help.

And drink plenty of water to keep your skin hydrated. You can visibly see the difference in your skin when you drink enough water.

STRENGTHEN YOUR LUNGS

The most important thing to do to strengthen your lungs is not to smoke and not to breathe secondhand smoke on a regular basis. Cigarette smoking is the number one cause of lung damage. And when lungs are damaged, they don't do a good job of expelling other toxic chemicals you are exposed to.

And take care to avoid indoor and outdoor air pollution that may damage your lungs.

On the positive side, take one hundred deep breaths every day. If that's too difficult, break it up into sets of however many you can do and work up. Doing deep breathing regularly can help your lungs flush out toxics, as well as stimulate your lymph system.

Get plenty of fresh air and outdoor exercise, such as brisk walking. In addition to other benefits of regular exercise, as your lungs inflate and deflate when you breathe hard, they become stronger and more able to function. I make a point to take a walk outdoors in fresh air at least thirty minutes a day (which means it doesn't happen every day, but if I say three times a week, it will be two, so I say every day and it's five).

Breathe steam. Turn on a hot shower and close the bathroom door to make steam, or breathe over a pot of steaming water. Be sure to use filtered water so you are not breathing in toxic chlorine or chloramines in the steam. Get a shower filter.

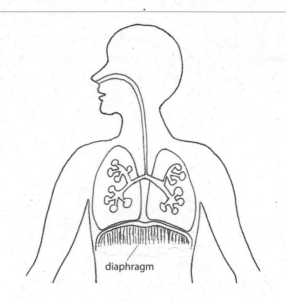

diaphragm

HOW TO BREATHE DEEPLY

Sit in a comfortable position with your hands on your knees. Relax your shoulders. Begin by slowly exhaling all the air from your lungs; draw in your diaphragm to help your lungs deflate. At the end of your breath, pause for a moment, then inhale slowly, allowing the air to expand your diaphragm.

How You Can Remove Toxic Chemicals from Your Body

While toxic chemicals can be eliminated by passing through your body's detox organs, there are also methods by which you can remove toxic chemicals from your body more directly.

Your body's detox system first removes the toxic chemicals that most recently came into your body. When, and only when, those chemicals are removed will it begin to work on the chemicals it has previously stored in your body. If you keep adding new chemicals to your body through everyday exposures, your body will never get around to removing the stored chemicals.

The following methods will work even if you do nothing else, but the best results will come from reducing toxic exposures, supporting your detox system, and strengthening your detox organs as well.

There are many products on the market now that claim to "remove toxins." The following are some tried-and-true methods for removing toxic chemicals from your body, which will help relieve your body's toxic burden. (And I will just say again: Because your individual body has its own needs, you may need to try different detox methods and products to find those which are best for you.)

DETOX FOODS

Garlic, cilantro, and chlorella are widely known to detox a variety of neurotoxicants, including heavy metals, biotoxins, man-made industrial toxics (including dioxin, phthalates, formaldehyde, insecticides, PCBs, and others), food preservatives and colors, fluoride, parabens, and others.

Some practitioners use large amounts of these foods for supervised detoxes to remove toxics quickly; however, you can use these three foods in your normal diet to gently benefit from their specific detox properties.

Garlic

Garlic contains numerous sulfur components that oxidize mercury, cadmium, and lead, making these metals water-soluble. This makes it easier for your body to excrete these metals.

Garlic also has many other benefits. It boosts the ability of your white blood cells to fight off bacterial infection, strengthens the cells of your immune system, reduces blood pressure and cholesterol levels, controls free radicals, and more.

Whole cloves of garlic need to be sliced, chopped, pressed or grated, cooked, or chewed to stimulate the garlic's healing properties.

I like to use the back of a fork to mash a raw garlic clove with a little Himalayan or sea salt into a paste in the bottom of my wooden salad

ROASTED GARLIC

Preheat the oven to 400 degrees.

Peel away the outer layers of the garlic bulb skin, leaving the skins of the individual cloves intact.

With a knife, cut off a bit of the top of each bulb, enough to expose each individual clove of garlic (remove garlic bits from paper skin and save for another recipe), and put the heads in a baking dish.

Drizzle with a little olive oil.

Bake for 30 to 35 minutes, or until the cloves feel soft when pressed.

Use a small fork or your fingers to pull or squeeze the roasted garlic cloves out of their skin.

Roasted garlic adds a rich flavor to any dish.

bowl before I make my salad. Then I add olive oil and other dressing ingredients and mix the dressing right in the bowl. This cuts the harshness of the garlic flavor and makes it easier to eat garlic raw.

I also love roasted garlic, which is very easy to make.

Cilantro (Chinese Parsley)

Cilantro is known to bind to mercury, cadmium, lead, aluminum, and other heavy metals, making it easier for your body to excrete these toxic metals through your kidneys. Removing these metals from your body reduces your overall body burden, leaving your detox organs free to remove other incoming chemicals.

A hospital in Japan, run by a Dr. Omura, was doing a study on heavy-metal poisoning with one hundred patients. One day, for no apparent reason, the patients suddenly started to pass heavy metals in their urine.

The doctors looked around for the cause of this. It turned out there was a new cook who served soup before all meals. In every bowl of soup he added "Vietnamese parsley," otherwise known as cilantro.

All metals were removed with the cilantro.

To detox your body using cilantro, the recommended amount is to take ¼ cup of *fresh* packed cilantro stems and leaves once daily for one to three weeks, along with Pascalite clay, 1 to 2 teaspoons in water three times daily. The clay helps to move the metal-laden cilantro through your intestines.

Dr. Omura also discovered that his patients suffered from fewer colds and less flu after removing the heavy metals because it seems

CILANTRO PESTO

1 cup packed fresh cilantro leaves
6 tablespoons olive oil
1 clove garlic
½ cup almonds, cashews, or other nuts
1 tablespoon lemon juice
Himalayan or sea salt to taste

Blend the cilantro and olive oil in a blender, add other ingredients to make a nice smooth paste.

MINT AND CILANTRO CHUTNEY

1 cup mint leaves
½ cup cilantro leaves
1 tablespoon fresh ginger, chopped
½ lime, juiced, plus more to taste
About ¼ cup water
Salt and freshly ground black pepper
1 tablespoon olive oil
1 teaspoon brown mustard seeds

Whiz together in blender or food processor.

A friend of mine makes a wonderful tomato salsa, to which she just adds a lot of cilantro. If you don't like the taste of cilantro, you can take a cilantro tincture.

that viruses and bacteria like to congregate in organs contaminated by heavy metals. His patients also had fewer herpes outbreaks after removing these heavy metals.

Cilantro leaves are commonly used in Mexican and Asian cooking. It is easy to grow in a flower pot. A few leaves as a garnish probably won't make much of a difference to your detox system, but if you can eat a significant amount on a regular basis, it can probably do some good.

Chlorella

Chlorella is a blue-green algae whole-food supplement. It also is known to bind to heavy metals, including cadmium, uranium, and lead, making it easier for your body to excrete them.

Chlorella is also a great supplement for vegetarians and vegans who want proteins and B vitamins from a nonanimal source.

Chlorella is about 60 percent protein and is considered to be a "complete protein" because it contains all the essential amino acids your body needs.

When choosing a brand of chlorella, it's important to choose one with a "broken cell wall." It's the cell wall that binds with the heavy metals. If you swallow the cell intact, it will not bind to the metals.

SWEAT

Sweat is the method used by your skin to remove poisons and wastes from your body. You can encourage your body to sweat by exercising, wearing warm clothing, using hot packs, sitting in the sun, taking hot showers, and other methods.

Though by itself sweat is not a major route of excretion of toxic chemicals, when accelerated by rigorous use of a sauna, sweat becomes a very effective method for removing toxic chemicals from your body.

Using various means to encourage sweat as a method of purification is a practice that goes back to ancient times and is found among most peoples around the world. The oldest known medical document, the Ayurveda, written in 568 B.C., considered sweating so important to health that it prescribed the sweat bath and thirteen other methods of inducing sweat.

The Roman steam bath, the Finnish *savusauna*, the Russian *banya*, the Native American sweat lodge, the Moroccan hammam—all have been used throughout history to induce sweat for body purification and restoration.

When you sit in a sweat bath, heat sensitive nerve endings produce acetylcholine, a chemical which alerts the eccrine sweat glands embedded in your skin all over your body (the sweat glands in your armpits actually don't respond to heat, they are activated by emotions). Eccrine sweat is clear and odorless; its chief function is to cool your body by evaporation.

During a fifteen-minute sauna, about two pints of sweat is excreted, depending upon the individual. This is about the amount the body generates naturally every day. It will also cause your body to excrete the same amount of heavy metals that your kidney would excrete in twenty-four hours.

Different types of sweat baths create different effects in your body, depending on the temperature and humidity of the air.

By far, the most recommended heat source for removing toxic chemicals from the body is a sauna.

There are doctors who administer sauna treatments specifically for the removal of toxic chemicals from the body. These are largely based on a sauna program developed by L. Ron Hubbard in the 1970s for the purpose of enabling drug addicts to detox drugs out of their bodies. This program, known as the Purification Rundown, proved to be very successful and is still in use today, around the world, for the purpose of removing drug residues from the body.

Shortly after the program was published in Mr. Hubbard's book *Clear Body, Clear Mind* in 1990, medical doctors realized that the method could be used to rid the body of many other types of chemicals, thereby restoring health from many diseases. Scientific studies show that this specific sauna program can remove phthalates and other plasticizers, PCBs, dioxins, pesticides, and other toxic chemicals.

The original Purification Rundown was designed to rid a body of drug and chemical residues to free an individual spiritually, not as a medical treatment, but it is a very effective body detox. It requires a commitment of time and money: five hours a day (for two to twelve weeks), exercise, vitamins, and about $1,500. The routine involves running to liberate toxic substances from body tissues and sweating in the sauna to release impurities from the body through the pores of the skin. But it is very effective. You can actually smell the toxic chemicals pouring out of bodies with the sweat. I personally know people who have done it with excellent results.

Doctors who use sauna for medical treatment usually give a thirty-day program for initial detox and then recommend patients buy their own saunas and continue to use them for life. This is about a $4,000 investment for the sauna, not including the cost of the doctor's detox program.

Saunas work. They are expensive, time-consuming, and tough to get through, but totally worth doing, if you can. They are the standard recommended treatment for people with multiple chemical sensitivities at the Environmental Health Center in Dallas, where individuals with the most difficult cases have gone for several decades.

For more information on saunas for detox, read *Clear Body, Clear Mind* by L. Ron Hubbard and *Detoxify or Die* by Sherry A. Rogers, M.D.

ACTIVATED LIQUID ZEOLITE

As I explained at the beginning of this chapter, this is what I take to remove toxic chemicals from my body.

Activated liquid zeolite is a very simple form of chelation therapy.

Chelators attract and hold heavy metals in the blood, making it easier for your body to excrete them through your kidneys.

Traditional chelation involves use of acid-based chelating agents such as EDTA, DMSA, and DMPS, administered intravenously while sitting in a doctor's office for four hours, three times a week. Twenty to forty sessions are required, costing thousands of dollars. And these chemical agents have no preference of attraction. They can just as easily remove calcium and other essential nutrients from your body along with mercury or lead.

Activated liquid zeolite also attracts and holds heavy metals in your blood making it easier for your body to excrete them through your kidneys, but it does so using simple tasteless, colorless, odorless drops you can take at home, at an affordable price, *without* also removing essential nutrients.

Zeolites are natural minerals with a unique, complex crystalline structure, made by volcanoes. The clinoptilolite zeolite molecule is shaped like a honeycomb, full of cavities and channels. Because zeolite carries a natural negative (–) charge, all of the positively charged (+) heavy metals, toxins, and harmful chemicals bond with the zeolite and are flushed out through the urine within six to eight hours.

Activated liquid zeolite can remove a wide variety of toxic substances from your body, including:

* Heavy metals, in this order: mercury, lead, tin, cadmium, arsenic, aluminum, antimony, nickel, then others
* Radioactive metals like cesium and strontium 90

As the free heavy metals are removed from the body, toxicants sequestered in fat cells and bones are pulled out so that, gradually, the toxic body burden is reduced.

Activated liquid zeolite does not directly bind to toxic chemicals, such as pesticides, herbicides, endocrine disruptors and dioxins; however, by reducing the toxic load to the liver, the liver becomes more able to remove these other chemicals using your body's own detoxification process.

Dr. Gabriel Cousens, M.D., did a study of sixty patients. He has worked with many patients over several decades, using juice and live foods for detox. Still, he highly recommends a specific brand of activated liquid zeolite (see my website www.debradetox.com for the exact brand) and uses it as a supplement to other detox methods and live food diets.

The protocol for Dr. Cousens's study consisted of a one-week green juice fast with liquid zeolite, 15 drops, four times a day. The toxics tested were heavy metals, radioactive materials, pesticides, and Teflon.

Here are the results of toxics removed in *one week*:

	LIVER	BREAST	BRAIN
Toxins found in 60 people BEFORE	845	876	875
Toxins found in 60 people AFTER	88	115	124
Toxins found per person BEFORE	14.1	14.6	14.6
Toxins found per person AFTER	1.5	1.9	2.1
Percentage removed	90%	87%	86%

The four patients who continued the green juice fasting with activated liquid zeolite for *two weeks* went down to zero toxins, a 100 percent removal rate. (It is not necessary to do the green juice fast to achieve results with activated liquid zeolite.)

I've tried a lot of detox products over the years, and activated liquid zeolite has been not only the most effective for me but also the easiest to take. The drops are crystal clear and flavorless, and can be placed in water or any food or beverage.

Liquid zeolite has "Generally Recognized as Safe (GRAS)" status from the FDA. You can take it every day. Even pregnant women, nursing mothers, and infants can take it.

One thing health care professionals I've talked to like about activated liquid zeolite is that it removes toxic substances from the body even if your detox organs—kidneys, liver, and intestines—are not up to par. It's a way to start reducing the toxic load on your body that is simple and easy.

I initially started taking activated liquid zeolite because I wanted to remove toxic chemicals that were already in my body. I continue to take it every day to help my body eliminate the new toxics I am continuously exposed to out in the world.

Living in today's world, where we are exposed to so many toxic chemicals, it is vitality important to keep your body's ability to detox in top shape. Your health depends on it.

For more information on activated liquid zeolite and detox, visit my website www.detox.com.

Life After Toxics

An ounce of prevention is worth a pound of cure.

—TRADITIONAL PROVERB

IFE AFTER TOXICS. I know that sounds like there is some toxic-free land over the rainbow somewhere or a new era when toxics are a thing of the past. Well, there is. There is actually a whole world of toxic-free possibilities. Not everything is toxic.

For most people, stepping out of the world of toxics means choosing a less toxic or toxic-free product instead of a toxic one. But there are more choices. You could make products yourself that are toxic-free—such as cleaning products, beauty products, and pest controls—and you could step outside the box altogether and live in harmony with nature with sustainable practices, doing things like growing your own organic food and producing your own renewable energy.

A new culture is already emerging where the intent is to sustain life. Many people around the world are already working on new technologies, rethinking industry, and discovering how to utilize the powers of nature to provide for our human needs in a way that supports and continues life. Toxic chemicals do not sustain life and so they are being phased out. There are enough people now in the world that understand this and are taking action that it *will* happen. Maybe not as fast as we might like, and maybe not without a struggle, but toxic chemicals *are* on their way out. You can help by choosing to be toxic-free.

I live in a toxic-free home and have a toxic-free body, so experiencing harm from toxics is, for me, a thing of the past. And my life after toxics is far better than it was when toxic chemicals ruled my health and my life.

While being exposed to toxics, my body was very sick, I couldn't think clearly, I was depressed, and I didn't have much of a life. I couldn't have a life: my body was too sick to do anything, and I was confined to my house, because everywhere I went, there were toxic chemicals that made me sick. The ravages of toxics kept me from doing the things I wanted to do.

Now, being free from toxics, I am healthy, active, and enjoy relationships. I have work that I love and participate in community activities with my friends. I can express my creativity and enjoy my spirituality. I travel, speak to groups, and appear on radio and television. My body is able and healthy, my mind is clear, and I have the freedom to do whatever I want—all because my body and mind are now unencumbered by the effects of toxic chemicals. And I know exactly what I need to do to keep toxic chemicals from being a problem for me.

The difference is not that the world has changed. There are still toxic chemicals all around. The difference is that *I* have changed.

I chose to be toxic-free and live this every day.

I consider getting sick from toxic chemical exposure to be one of the greatest blessings of my life, because I had the opportunity to become aware that toxic chemicals do exist in the world and can harm my body. That awareness gave me the power to be able to do something about it and not be a victim. Now you have that power too.

The key is to focus on creating health, and that requires a bit of a change in how we think. In our culture, the tendency is not to do something right to begin with but rather to do something that doesn't quite work and then find a solution to the problem.

Here's an example. My new refrigerator makes a little beeping sound when I don't fully shut the door. This is touted as a great energy-saving feature—one that my old refrigerator didn't have. Except for one thing: the old refrigerator didn't need the beeping sound because all I had to do was push the door in the direction of being closed and it would fall shut all by itself. This new door I have to push all the way shut. It won't close fully on its own.

The way we take care of our bodies is similar. We don't pay much attention to proper care and maintenance in the first place; instead, we eat whatever, drink whatever, expose our bodies to toxic chemicals, fail to exercise, and fail to sleep. Then, when our bodies fail to function properly, we turn to expensive industrialized health care.

Our bodies are designed to be healthy when properly maintained within the system of nature they belong to. If we do the steps that result in health, health will be the result.

In today's world, the first step to health is removing toxic industrial chemicals from our bodies, our homes, and the environment, because toxic chemicals work against the life-support processes of nature. Removing toxic chemicals allows the rejuvenating processes naturally inherent in our bodies to work.

I'm not fighting toxics. I'm choosing health and taking action accordingly, and toxics just aren't part of that. I just eliminated toxics from my life. And they can be eliminated in the world if each of us just chooses not to use them. It really is that simple.

Do you think that manufacturers would make toxic products if none of us purchased them? The answer is no. Already major manufacturers of toxic products are starting to offer less toxic products. I've talked to some of them. And you know what they say? *They would offer more toxic-free products if consumers would buy them!* So it really is in our hands. We consumers have the power to make a toxic-free world by refusing to purchase products that contain toxic chemicals and instead choosing to purchase products that are toxic-free

What it all actually comes down to is each one of us choosing to be toxic-free and then taking the actions to do so.

Doing the right thing that results in supporting life is a personal choice. We wouldn't need laws at all if each individual simply took responsibility and made personal choices that led in the direction of sustaining life. Laws are only necessary when we don't do this. And right now, we do need them.

There are toxic chemicals in the world, lots of them, all around you. You may not have control over all of them. But how they affect *you* and your loved ones is *your choice.*

You get to choose if you want your body to be sick or healthy.

You get to choose if you are exposed to toxics or not.

You get to choose how you will support your body's detox system or not and whether or not you will remove toxic chemicals from your body.

It's all your choice.

CHOOSE TO BE TOXIC-FREE.

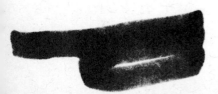

APPENDIX A

How Toxics Affect Your Body Systems

HAVE BEEN STUDYING and writing about the health effects of toxic chemicals on the human body for three decades. In the past, particular chemicals would be associated with a list of symptoms, such as headache, dizziness, and the like.

Today, there is ample evidence that specific toxic chemicals affect whole body systems, and so we speak of chemicals that are, for example, "endocrine disruptors" that affect the entire endocrine system, causing a whole constellation of body conditions and symptoms.

I've included this appendix in this book because we need to think of our toxic exposures in terms of how they impact our body systems. Yet, most of us really aren't aware of the systems that run the functions of our bodies. I certainly wasn't. I knew, for example, that I had an endocrine system, but I didn't know how it worked or what could happen to my health if my endocrine system was damaged by toxic chemicals. I gained a whole different perspective on my health when I started

177

looking at my body systems and their functions. I now understand what my body is doing when I lift my arm or put a bite of food in my mouth, and greatly appreciate all the services my body provides to me, now that I am aware of them.

In the world of toxicology, there are twelve basic types of toxicants, each of which cause illness in a specific body system (although today I am seeing more and more new toxicant types being coined that refer to specific body conditions, such as asthmatogens, which can cause asthma, and even obesogens, which can cause obesity!). As you read about each one, you'll see that virtually all of the symptoms, conditions, and illnesses for which people take over-the-counter and prescription drugs can be caused by exposure to toxic chemicals. I've included both the scientific and common terminology so you will know what terms to use if you want to do more research on any of the toxicants or body systems.

Even though toxicants are classified by individual body systems according to their target organs, it is important to remember, too, that all *body systems work together*. The body is one unified whole, so when one body system falters, the other body systems start falling like dominoes. In reality, a toxicant that harms one body system harms the whole body.

As an example, just to move your body, a bone needs a muscle to move it. But a muscle needs blood vessels to bring nutrients and oxygen for energy and to carry away wastes. And muscles need nerves to bring a message from the brain that says, "Move that muscle." And muscles need the digestive system to process food so the muscle has fuel. And on and on. Every part of your body is interconnected with every other part, and they all operate together in one system. All for one, and one for all.

In this section, I list some symptoms and illnesses that can result from exposure to toxicants, along with some of the specific toxicants that cause those health effects. For more information on specific toxicants, their related health effects, and how and where you might be exposed to these substances, visit www.knowtoxicsnow.com.

Here is an overview of the damages that can happen to your body systems when you are exposed to toxic chemicals. Fortunately, they are also the conditions that can be prevented and healed when you choose to be toxic-free.

Your Cells

The cell is the basic structural unit of all living organisms. A cell contains a nucleus, along with other functional parts, within a membrane that encloses the cell and regulates the exchange of material between the inside of the cell and its surrounding environment.

Within the nucleus of every cell is deoxyribonucleic acid (DNA), which contains the genetic instructions used in the development and functioning of your body. DNA is often compared to a set of blueprints, like a recipe or a code, since it contains the instructions needed to construct other components of cells. The DNA segments that carry this genetic information are called genes, and genes are organized into long structures called chromosomes.

Genes are inherited from your parents. It takes thirty to forty thousand genes to make up your twenty-three pairs of chromosomes. Every cell in your body contains its own twenty-three pairs of chromosomes that control how that cell grows and works.

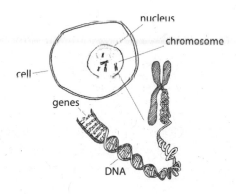

DNA is important to all cells, and to every living organism, because:

- It passes genetic information to new cells during the process of cell division.

- It passes genetic information from one generation to the next during reproduction.
- It provides all the genetic information needed to carry out the major functions of a cell.

Your body can do nothing without DNA.

Processes that keep your body alive are going on continuously in your body's cells, day and night. To maintain these life processes, an ongoing exchange of substances occurs between the cell and its surrounding environment. Nutrients, oxygen, salts, hormones, and other substances enter the cell, and carbon dioxide, water, and waste materials are discharged from the cell. All these substances, coming in and going out, pass through the cell membrane.

HOW TOXIC CHEMICALS HARM YOUR CELLS

Just as nutrients, oxygen, and other substances come through the cell membrane, so, too, can toxic chemicals.

Genotoxicants are substances that harm the genetic information contained in the DNA of every cell in your body.

When a gene is altered in some way due to exposure to genotoxicants, it doesn't work properly and can give wrong instructions.

Genotoxicants are often classified as:

- **mutagens:** cause a permanent change in the DNA of a cell
- **carcinogens:** cause a damaged cell to divide at an uncontrolled rate so that a cancer tumor develops
- **terotogens:** cause structural or functional "birth defects" in the developing embryo or fetus, growth retardation, or death of the embryo or fetus when the mother or father is exposed to the chemical before or during pregnancy

These are all genotoxicants because they all alter DNA.

There are thousands of chemicals that can damage DNA—too many to list here. They include tobacco smoke (direct and secondhand), alcoholic beverages and other sources of ethyl alcohol, solvents, pesticides, food coloring, dioxin, car exhaust, lead, and many other chemicals we are exposed to every day.

A study of ancient human remains done at Manchester University in the United Kingdom shows that cancer is a man-made disease caused by toxic chemical pollution and eating industrialized food. There is virtually nothing in the natural environment that can cause cancer. After studying Egyptian mummies, fossils, and classical literature, little evidence of cancer was found. Even the study of thousands of Neanderthal bones produced only one example of a possible cancer. The first reports in scientific literature of distinctive cancer tumors only occurred in the past two hundred years.

Further evidence that cancer is a man-made illness comes from the tiny kingdom of Hunza, nestled between Pakistan, India, and China. These people never contract cancer or suffer from heart disease if they eat their native diet. Recently, however, a road has been built into Hunza and Western food has been brought in. Now there is cancer in Hunza.

The same is true of Eskimos living on the polar ice, eating their native diet, which consists mostly of wild game and wild berries. They have no cancer, either.

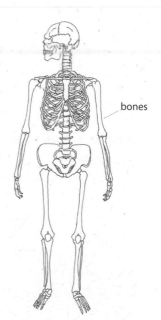

bones

Even more important to consider is that when you damage your own DNA with exposure to toxic chemicals, you are also compromising future generations as well. Genetic information gets passed on, whether healthy or mutated. Already we are seeing that younger generations are less healthy than grandparents born and raised prior to the explosion of toxic chemicals in consumer products.

Your Skeletal System

Your skeletal system is made up of all the bones in your body and the joints between them.

Bones make up the skeleton framework of your body, giving muscles and organs a place to attach themselves. The bones of your skeleton give your body shape and posture. Without your spine (backbone), you would be unable to stand erect.

Bones also shield the softer parts of your body that are essential to being alive:

- Your skull protects your brain.
- Your spine protects all the nerves in your spinal column.
- Your ribs make a protective cage around your lungs, heart, and liver.

Some bones also make your blood cells. The bones in your body produce approximately 2.6 million red blood cells per second to replace the cells that are routinely being destroyed by your liver, so healthy bones are absolutely vital.

Bones, together with muscles, make up your musculoskeletal system (also called the locomotor system), which gives your body the ability to move. Made up of the muscular system and skeletal system, your musculoskeletal system's muscles and bones work together to give your body form, support, stability, and movement.

The points where bones connect to other bones are called joints.

HOW TOXIC CHEMICALS HARM YOUR SKELETAL SYSTEM

Skeletal toxicants cause adverse effects to the bones and joints of your skeletal system.

Bone disorders and their causes include:

- bone cancer (radium and pesticides)
- osteoporosis (aluminum, cadmium, fluoride, and tobacco smoke)
- fluorosis (fluoride)
- delayed growth (alcoholic beverages and other sources of ethyl alcohol, lead, mercury, PCBs, and toluene)

- skeletal malformations, including limb reduction, two or more fingers fused together, and more than five fingers or toes (ethyl alcohol, arsenic)

Joint problems include:

- rheumatoid arthritis (tobacco smoke)
- gout (lead)

Parental exposure to pesticides has been associated with a three- to fourfold risk of skeletal malformations in their children.

Your Muscular System

Your muscular system is made up of all the muscles in your body and the connective tissues between them.

The primary function of muscles is to provide postural stability for your body so you can stand up.

Muscles, attached to bones, make up your musculoskeletal system (also called locomotor system), which gives your body the ability to move. Through the contraction and relaxation of muscles, you can move your body in many ways:

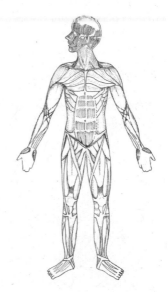

- Limb muscles allow you to walk and exert force.
- Finger muscles allow you to hold, move, and manipulate objects.
- The diaphragm muscle causes your lungs to expand so you can breathe.
- The pharynx muscle allows you to swallow.
- Tongue and lip muscles allow you to take food into your body and speak (and kiss!).

Involuntary functions (muscle movements you cannot control) include:

- propulsion of substances through body passages, such as food through your digestive tract, blood through your vessels, and lymph fluid through lymph vessels
- expulsion of stored substances, such as bile from your gallbladder
- regulation of the size of openings, such as the pupils of your eyes to adjust to light
- regulation of the diameter of tubes, such as blood vessels

Because of the amount of muscle mass on your body (muscles make up 40 percent of your body's total weight), they are your body's main source of heat generation. Muscles also help to regulate the body's temperature, keeping it constant.

Connective tissue is a type of tissue made up of fibers forming a framework and support structure for body tissues and organs. It is the material between the cells of the body that gives tissues form and strength.

HOW TOXIC CHEMICALS HARM YOUR MUSCULAR SYSTEM

Muscular toxicants affect the ability of your muscles to function.

Because the muscular system holds your body upright, enables movement, and generates heat, damage to muscles can be devastating not only to the muscles themselves but also to the body's entire ability to function. Muscular system disorders are often very painful and result in physical impairments, such as an inability to walk.

There was a time in my life when my body was suffering from hypothyroidism, the result of toxic chemical exposure. I control that condition today with a natural thyroid supplement, but at the time, my body was rapidly declining due to an insufficient amount of thyroid hormone. As my condition worsened, muscles throughout my body would begin to spasm when I moved them, to the point where I could barely swallow even a sip of water. Fortunately, I got the right treatment before I went into a coma, and my muscle function was restored. But I certainly learned to appreciate my muscles from that experience.

Disorders of the muscular system known to be associated with toxic chemical exposure include:

- cerebral palsy (mercury)
- multiple sclerosis (pesticides, solvents)
- spastic muscles (mercury)

Your Skin

Your skin is part of your body's integumentary system, made up of multiple layers of skin, plus glands, hair, and nails.

Your integumentary system (which literally means "to cover") is the largest organ system of your body, comprising 12 to 15 percent of your body weight and having a surface area of one to two square yards.

The soft outer covering of your skin provides important functions to your body:

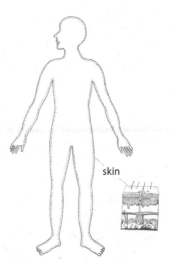

skin

- It provides a layer of protection from pathogens, physical abrasions, and radiation from the sun, and between the internal environment of your body and the external environment.
- It maintains a constant body temperature via the acts of sweating (to cool your body down) or shivering (to warm your body up).
- Sensation for touch, pain, and heat is provided by nerve endings.
- It enables the metabolism of vitamin D.
- It facilitates the excretion of salts and small amounts of toxic chemicals with the production of sweat.

HOW TOXIC CHEMICALS HARM YOUR SKIN

Toxic chemicals that damage your skin are called "dermatotoxicants."

As the barrier between your body and its surrounding environment, your skin is exposed to many toxic chemicals in cosmetics, household products, medications, tap water, and other everyday products.

Skin irritation and skin corrosion are immediate toxic effects resulting from direct skin exposure to a toxic substance. The difference is skin irritation is reversible damage and skin corrosion is irreversible damage, such as when lye in drain cleaner eats through the skin. Rashes are often reactions to toxic exposures, as well as swelling and increased blood flow through dilated blood vessels.

Skin sensitization is an allergic reaction to a particular substance that results in the development of skin inflammation and itchiness. In contrast to skin irritation, the skin becomes increasingly reactive to the substance as it is exposed over and over.

Phototoxicity is when the skin becomes very sensitive to light. It can be caused by rubbing toxic chemicals on the skin. Phototoxicity causes sunburn, redness of the skin, blisters, darkening of the skin, shedding of layers of skin, and other skin problems.

More serious skin problems include hives, eczema, and skin cancer.

Your skin can also become disturbed as a result of attempting to expel toxic substances from your body. A friend of mine who works with cancer patients daily sees clients with skin breakouts as a result of chemotherapy.

Body odor can also be an indicator that the body is trying to get rid of toxic substances. I once met a man whose body reeked of a toxic solvent.

Your Nervous System

Your nervous system controls and coordinates all of your body functions. It has two parts: the central nervous system (CNS) is made of your brain and spinal cord, and the peripheral nervous system (PNS) is the network of nerves that run throughout your body.

Your brain is the command center of your body. Your spinal cord is a bundle of nerves that run up and down your spine, speeding messages to nerves that carry them back and forth between your brain and every part of your body.

There are many viewpoints as to what exactly is doing the thinking and feeling within a human organism. Scientists who study only the physical body tell us it is the brain; others say there is an invisible mind made of energy independent of the body; and there is also the viewpoint that we are spiritual beings by nature, without form or substance, existing beyond space and time. Whatever your orientation as to the origin of thought and feeling, the brain functions as the central command post for communications throughout the body.

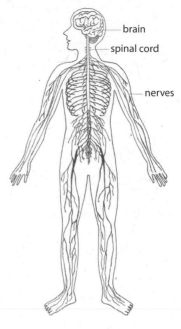

brain

spinal cord

nerves

Certainly, science has shown that different areas of the brain, when stimulated, evoke specific responses. Different parts of the brain govern reasoning, planning, speech, balance, coordination, movement, emotions, problem solving, orientation, recognition, memory, perception, and recognition of sensory stimuli.

The brain stem is in charge of all the functions your body needs to stay alive, like breathing air, digesting food, and circulating blood. Part of the brain stem's job is to control your involuntary muscles, like telling your heart to pump more blood when you're walking fast or your stomach to start digesting your dinner. The brain stem also sorts through the millions of messages that the brain and the rest of the body send back and forth through the nervous system.

Your physical senses are part of your nervous system. Sensory nerves in your eyes, ears, mouth, nose, and skin gather information from the environment and send it back to the brain. Each sensor can detect only the sensation it is supposed to detect. Your brain combines all the sensations it is receiving to get the whole picture.

HOW TOXIC CHEMICALS HARM YOUR NERVOUS SYSTEM

Neurotoxicants are so called because they are toxic to your nervous system.

Some of the more common neurotoxicants include aluminum, acetone, pesticides, ammonia, benzene, ethylene glycol, fluoride, formaldehyde, lead, and other common chemicals we are exposed to every day.

Some of the adverse effects of neurotoxicants specific to the nervous system include:

- headache
- fatigue
- emotional upsets
- inability to think clearly
- impaired sensory perception
- disorientation
- slowness
- fever and chills
- weight loss or gain
- rash
- insomnia
- confusion
- change in personality
- extreme fatigue
- memory loss
- loss of coordination
- difficulty speaking or understanding what is being said
- staring into space
- twitching
- episodes of bizarre behavior
- dizziness
- ringing in the ears
- visual disturbances
- tingling or numbness
- irritability
- behavioral changes

- muscle weakness
- rapid heartbeat
- aches and pains
- autism
- ADD/ADHD, hyperactivity
- Alzheimer's
- brain cancer
- dementia
- Parkinson's disease

Because the nerves regulate functions throughout the entire body, having toxic chemicals damaging your nervous system affects every function.

As only one example, all of us have cancer cells in our body right now. Every day, each of our bodies make cancer cells. However, if your immune system organs are functioning normally, these cancer cells will be destroyed before they turn into tumors. But what controls your immune system? Your nervous system!

Because your nervous system controls every single cell, organ, and gland in your body, if you protect your nervous system from neurotoxicants, the rest of your body will do well too.

The number of chemicals known to be neurotoxic that we are exposed to in everyday consumer products has been estimated to be well over one thousand, but the exact number cannot be determined because data is lacking for the vast majority of chemicals suspected to be neurotoxic. Meanwhile, products containing these chemicals continue to be sold. Just a few examples of common products that contain neurotoxicants are perfume and scented products, permanent-ink markers, and tap water.

Your Circulatory System

Your cardiovascular system (also called the circulatory system) is all about delivering oxygen and nutrients throughout your body via a complex network of arteries, veins, and other vessels—more than sixty thousand miles of vessels in all. If you laid all your blood vessels end to end, you could wrap them around the earth at the equator twice and still have a piece long enough to stretch from New York City to Sydney, Australia.

This vital role of nutrient and oxygen delivery depends on the continuous and controlled movement of blood through thousands of miles of capillaries that permeate every tissue and reach every cell in your body. Through the capillary walls, nutrients and other essential materials pass from capillary blood into fluids surrounding the cells as waste products are removed.

The muscles of your heart squeeze and relax about seventy times per minute (if you are an adult) to pump your blood to every part of your body.

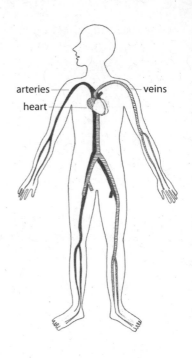

HOW TOXIC CHEMICALS HARM YOUR CIRCULATORY SYSTEM

Cardiotoxicants impair the function of your heart and blood. Since blood flows throughout your body, damage done by cardiotoxicants can be widespread.

Toxic exposures can have adverse effects on both the heart and blood vessels or the blood that flows within them.

The major heart problems caused by exposure to toxicants include:

- elevated blood pressure (lead, arsenic, carbon monoxide)
- hardening of the arteries (tobacco smoke, lead, arsenic, cadmium, carbon monoxide, mercury)
- abnormal heartbeat (arsenic, carbon monoxide, CFCs, dihalomethane, nitrates/nitrites, pesticides)
- deterioration of the function of the heart muscle (carbon monoxide, arsenic, lead, cadmium)

- heart attack (carbon monoxide, cyanide, dihalomethanes, nitrates/ nitrites, tobacco smoke—direct and secondhand)
- stroke (lead, air pollution, tobacco smoke—direct and secondhand)

Exposure to blood toxicants can:

- reduce the oxygen carrying capacity of red blood cells
- disrupt important immunological processes carried out by white blood cells
- induce cancer

Your Immune System

Your immune system is composed of biological structures and processes that protect your body from infectious disease. It identifies and kills bacteria, viruses, fungi, protozoa, parasites, and other harmful microorganisms (known collectively as "germs") and tumor cells. The different parts work together to keep germs out of your body and to attack and destroy any that do manage to get inside.

Your skin, which acts as a barrier to germs, is the first line of defense. Mucous membranes inside the nose, mouth, and eyes also act as barriers to germs.

The lymphatic system is a network of very small vessels that sends a clear fluid all through your body that collects germs and brings them back to lymph nodes, where they are filtered out and destroyed. The major parts of the lymph tissue are located in the bone marrow, spleen, thymus gland, lymph nodes, and tonsils. The heart, lungs, intestines, liver, and skin also contain lymphatic tissue. The spleen clears worn-out red blood cells and other foreign bodies from the bloodstream to help fight off infection.

But there are also many other mechanisms throughout your body that are constantly working to protect your body from harmful microorganisms. The gastrointestinal tract, for example, with a surface area the size of a football field, has its own lymphoid tissue to prevent pathogens present in ingested foods from entering into the bloodstream and lymph system.

HOW TOXIC CHEMICALS HARM YOUR IMMUNE SYSTEM

Immunotoxicants damage your immune system.

Immunotoxicants suppress the immune system's ability to respond adequately to invading agents, leaving the body open for any infectious-disease microorganisms to enter. In addition to the common cold and flu, infectious diseases include:

- candidiasis
- chicken pox
- cholera
- diarrhea
- hepatitis
- herpes
- HIV/AIDS
- Lyme disease
- malaria
- measles
- meningitis
- mumps
- pneumonia
- respiratory infections
- smallpox
- strep throat
- tuberculosis
- typhus
- venereal diseases

These are also called communicable diseases or transmissible diseases because they are passed from one person to another via germs. When your immune system is weak due to exposure to toxic chemicals, your body is more susceptible to any communicable disease.

A weak immune system can also make any other disease more severe.

Exposure to immunotoxicants can also cause autoimmune diseases, in which healthy tissue in the body is attacked by an immune system that fails to differentiate between substances and tissues normally in the body and foreign invaders. Some well-recognized autoimmune diseases are:

- celiac disease
- Crohn's disease
- Guillain-Barre syndrome
- Hashimoto's thyroiditis
- lupus
- psoriasis
- rheumatoid arthritis
- ulcerative colitis

As I stated in the Introduction, my own personal introduction to the world of toxics was through multiple chemical sensitivities (MCS), also caused by immunotoxicants. A person becomes sensitive through immune system damage caused by either a onetime dangerously high-level exposure (such as an industrial chemical spill or pesticide spraying) or continuous low-level exposure, as in modern homes and office buildings. Once the damage is done, all sorts of low-level exposures, such as to perfume or cleaning products, can cause symptoms. All sorts of symptoms are possible, including dizziness, fainting, itchy or burning eyes, runny or congested nose, dry throat, shortness of breath, asthma, upset stomach, diarrhea, menstrual problems, extreme fatigue, insomnia, memory lapses, poor concentration, depression, and behavioral changes.

Common allergens are also considered immunotoxicants, causing allergy symptoms such as asthma, stuffy nose, and anaphylactic shock.

Many years ago, when I worked in the office of an immunologist who practiced environmental medicine, we observed that food allergies would disappear in patients when we removed the toxic chemicals from their homes. Apparently food allergies are the result of toxic overload on the immune system. Perhaps other allergies are the result of toxic overload as well.

Some common immunotoxicants include vinyl chloride, benzene, copper, lead, mercury, naphthalene, pesticides, and solvents.

Your Excretory System

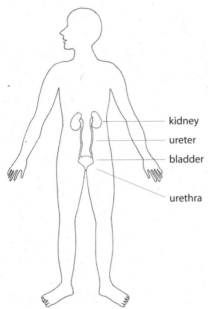

kidney
ureter
bladder

urethra

The excretory system of your body is composed of your kidneys and urinary system.

In traditional Chinese medicine, the kidney (of which there are two) is considered the most important organ in the body. It is the key organ involved in purifying the blood and the rejuvenating and recycling center for your body.

Every four minutes the total volume of blood in your body passes through and is "filtered" by the kidneys. This process not only removes excess, unnecessary, or dangerous materials from your body but also helps recycle nutrients carried in the blood, such as glucose, vitamins, minerals, and other important substances.

Your excretory system is responsible for the elimination of the waste products of cell metabolism. As your blood circulates, distributing oxygen and nutrients, it also collects wastes from every cell in your body. As your blood flows through your kidneys, they filter your blood to remove the collected wastes.

Every cell in your body depends on the function of your excretory system for the removal of liquid and gaseous wastes, so if the excretory system is compromised, the entire body can have health problems.

The kidneys filter the blood and produce urine, which is held in the bladder until it fills and empties through the urethra.

Other functions of the urinary system are:

- to maintain the volume and composition of body fluids within normal limits, including the production of urine
- to control red blood cell production
- to regulate blood pressure and volume
- to help maintain calcium for bones

Because of their vital role to the body, it's important to protect your kidneys.

HOW TOXIC CHEMICALS HARM YOUR EXCRETORY SYSTEM

Nephrotoxicants have adverse effects on your kidneys, ureter, or bladder.

Your kidneys are unusually susceptible to toxic exposures because of their role in filtering harmful substances from your blood. The more chemicals you are exposed to, the more damage you will do to your kidneys, making it even more difficult for your body to withstand toxic exposures.

Some of these toxicants cause immediate injury to your kidneys, while others produce long-term changes that can lead to end-stage kidney failure or cancer.

Some of the more common nephrotoxicants are carbon tetrachloride, trichloroethylene, chloroform, solvents, and the heavy metals cadmium, chromium, mercury, and lead.

Your Digestive System

Your digestive system (also called the gastrointestinal system) includes all the glands and organs in the entire digestive tract, from food going into your mouth to wastes coming out at the other end.

There is the digestive tract itself, through which the food moves, and other accessory digestive glands that assist digestion but are not part of the digestive tract, including the salivary glands, liver, gallbladder, and pancreas.

When you put food into your mouth and chew it up into small pieces, your body releases saliva to mix with the food so it can easily slide down the esophagus into the stomach. In your stomach, acid is mixed with the food to continue digestion.

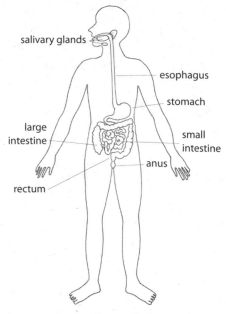

Next, the food is pushed into your small intestine, where enzymes are added to help with digestion. Most food is turned into very small particles, which are absorbed through the wall of the small intestine into the blood and sent via the blood to different parts of the body where they are needed. Undigested bits of food that can't be absorbed through the wall of the small intestine go down into the large intestine, where further digestion takes place. The large intestine also contributes to hydrating your body by absorbing water from the food you eat.

Everything that is now left over stays in the lowest part of the bowel, the rectum, until enough accumulates to trigger a release through the anus.

Metabolism is the breaking down of food into usable nutrients that are then used to repair and build your body. It begins in the digestive system, where enzymes break proteins down into amino acids, fats into fatty acids, and carbohydrates into simple sugars. These compounds are absorbed into the blood, which carries them to the cells.

After these compounds enter the cells, various chemical reactions occur to "metabolize" them. During these processes, the energy from these compounds can be released for use by the body or stored for future use in the liver, muscles, and body fat.

Metabolism brings nutrients and energy to every cell in the body, but it all starts in the digestive system.

HOW TOXIC CHEMICALS HARM YOUR DIGESTIVE SYSTEM

The gastrointestinal tract is primarily affected by toxic chemicals that are ingested by eating food and drinking beverages. These toxicants cause such symptoms as

- anorexia
- nausea
- vomiting
- abdominal cramps
- diarrhea
- cancer

Common gastrointestinal toxicants include food additives (such as preservatives, artificial colors and flavors, nitrites/nitrates), pesticides, water chlorination by-products, chromium, and solvents.

Your Liver

The liver is considered an organ of the digestive system because some of its functions aid digestion.

I am addressing it as a separate system because it performs many functions beyond digestion and because it is damaged by its own specific set of toxicants.

Your liver is the largest organ inside your body (your skin is the largest organ in your entire body).

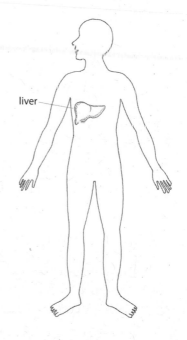

liver

Your liver's primary function is to aid in digestion and remove waste products and worn-out cells from your blood. Your liver:

- changes most of the food that you eat into molecules your body can use
- makes a digestive juice called bile (about a quart a day) that helps the body absorb fat from the gut into the bloodstream (stored in the gallbladder until the body needs some to digest fat and cholesterol)
- breaks down proteins into amino acids
- breaks down carbohydrates into glucose

The liver also performs more than five hundred other vital functions, including:

- getting rid of the materials that are of no use or are toxic
- storing fuel in the form of glucose and glycogen
- helping to keep blood sugar at the right levels
- storing vitamins A, D, K, and B_{12}
- producing cholesterol, a fat that your body needs for normal growth and health

But most important to our topic of toxics: your liver breaks down fat-soluble toxicants into a water-soluble form that your body can excrete (see Chapter 4).

HOW TOXIC CHEMICALS HARM YOUR LIVER

Toxic chemicals that cause adverse effects on your liver are called hepatotoxicants.

While your liver is the primary organ your body uses to remove fat-soluble toxicants, it is also one of the most susceptible to damage precisely because of its function as the body's principal site of metabolism. Most toxicants that come into the body end up in the liver.

The liver has a remarkable ability to regenerate, but still, large exposures to toxicants all at once or over time do cause damage, including:

- liver necrosis (cell death)
- cirrhosis of the liver
- hepatitis
- liver cancer

Probably the most common liver toxicant that does the most widespread damage is the alcohol in alcoholic beverages. In addition, some industrial chemicals that can damage the liver are chloroform, solvents, and carbon tetrachloride.

Your Respiratory System

The main job of your respiratory system is to bring fresh oxygen into your body and remove carbon dioxide and other waste gases. Without oxygen, your body cannot survive. After only three to four minutes without oxygen, your brain cells start to die.

In addition to exchanging carbon dioxide for fresh oxygen, your respiratory system protects your body from harmful substances (by coughing, sneezing, filtering, or swallowing them) and provides your sense of smell.

If you are an average adult, you take fifteen to twenty breaths a minute—more than twenty thousand breaths a day—bringing into your body whatever is in the surrounding air. Air comes into the body through the nose or mouth as you inhale and travels through the pharynx, trachea, and bronchi to the lungs. The lungs are so important to survival that they are completely protected from damage by the bones of your rib cage. Below your lungs, a large muscle called the diaphragm expands and contracts to get air in and out of the lungs.

Once the air is inside your lungs, oxygen from the air moves into the capillaries of the cardiovascular system. The red blood cells in all the tiny blood vessels then carry the blood to your heart, which pumps the oxygen-rich blood to every cell in your body.

As each red blood cell empties its load of oxygen, it picks up carbon dioxide from the cell and heads back to the lungs. There, the carbon dioxide is emptied into the air that leaves the body when you exhale through your nose or mouth.

HOW TOXIC CHEMICALS HARM YOUR RESPIRATORY SYSTEM

Respiratory toxicants cause damage to your respiratory system.

Because the delicate tissue of your lungs is directly connected to the outside environment, everything you inhale can affect your lungs. While each breathe brings life-giving oxygen into your body, that same breath can also bring in germs, smoke, dust, gases, and other pollutants that can cause damage to your airways and threaten the ability of your lungs to work properly.

Respiratory responses to toxic exposures can include a variety of acute and chronic lung conditions, including:

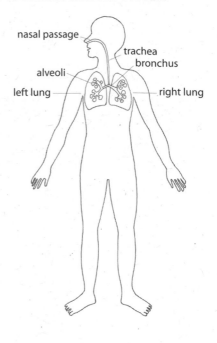

- local irritation resulting in coughing, sneezing, runny nose, and other nose and throat symptoms
- asthma
- chronic obstructive pulmonary disease (COPD), also known as emphysema, and chronic bronchitis
- pulmonary fibrosis
- lung cancer
- death by asphyxiation

Toxic exposures can also constrict the airways, resulting in not enough oxygen in your blood. When this happens, your entire body is affected.

Some common toxicants that produce respiratory effects include ammonia, chlorine, mercury, plastic fumes, all types of dusts and particles, and tobacco smoke (direct and secondhand).

Your Endocrine System

Like your nervous system, your endocrine system is a communi-cations system, influencing almost every cell, organ, and function of your body.

The endocrine system regulates such vital functions as mood, growth and development, production and utilization of insulin, rate of metabolism, intelligence and behavior, response to stress, as well as sexual development and behavior and reproductive processes.

Most of the functions of your body are triggered by the interaction between hormones and their receptor sites in the endocrine glands. Receptors are like locks; hormones and other molecules are like keys. The "keys" circulate through the body until they find the right "locks." When a hormone key is inserted into its correct receptor lock, a communication is made that regulates essential body functions.

These are the glands that make up the human endo-crine system:

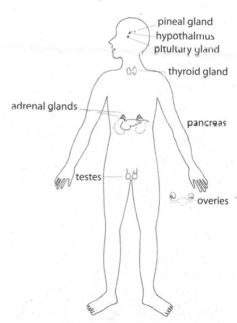

- **pituitary gland:** called the master gland; regulates all other glands
- **hypothalamus:** provides information sensed by the brain (such as environmental temperature, light exposure patterns, and feelings) to the pituitary, and is the link between the endocrine system and the nervous system

pineal gland
hypothalmus
pituitary gland
thyroid gland
adrenal glands
pancreas
testes
overies

- **thyroid:** controls the rate at which cells burn fuels from food to produce energy
- **parathyroids:** regulate the level of calcium in the blood
- **adrenal glands:** regulate mineral (including salt) and water balance in the body, the body's response to stress, metabolism, the immune system, and sexual development and function
- **pineal gland:** regulates sleep cycles
- **reproductive glands (ovaries and testes):** regulate sex and reproduction
- **pancreas:** maintains a steady level of glucose, or sugar, in the blood and keeps the body supplied with fuel to produce and maintain stores of energy

HOW TOXIC CHEMICALS HARM YOUR ENDOCRINE SYSTEM

Endocrine toxicants—also called endocrine disruptors—affect the endocrine system.

The problem with endocrine toxicants is that they can mimic hormones and enter the receptors, interfering with the body's ability to make its own natural connections. This can lead to health problems such as:

- thyroid dysfunction
- reproductive problems (including infertility, menopause symptoms, low sex drive, impotence, alterations in sexual behavior, and cancer of the reproductive organs)
- prostate enlargement
- bladder incontinence
- high blood pressure
- inability to lose weight
- gallbladder problems
- hair loss
- fatigue
- insomnia
- depression

- constipation
- diabetes mellitus

In the female reproductive system particularly, toxic chemicals known as xenoestrogens (literally, "foreign estrogens") interfere with the natural estrogens in a woman's body, leading to many reproductive problems.

Though I recovered from multiple chemical sensitivities many years ago, they were followed by ongoing thyroid problems, infertility, insomnia, adult-onset diabetes, high blood pressure, high cholesterol, fatigue, adrenal exhaustion, and problems losing weight. Attempts to improve these conditions by standard and alternative means were to no avail.

Then new research about endocrine disruptors began to appear and I began to see this constellation of health problems in a new light. *They are all—directly or indirectly— disorders of the endocrine system.* Understanding this and their connection to toxic chemical exposure, I was able to start handling these conditions.

According to the Endocrine Disruption Exchange (www.endo crinedisruption.com), to date, no chemical in use has been thoroughly tested for its endocrine disrupting effects. However, hundreds of sci entific studies have demonstrated endocrine impairment as the result of toxic chemicals such as pesticides, fungicides, herbicides, plastics, detergents, perfume, heavy metals (lead, mercury, cadmium, preservatives, and others). Hormones in birth control pills, in hormone replacement therapy, in our food supply, and even in natural foods such as soy can also alter our hormone connections.

APPENDIX B

/

Be Your Own Toxicologist

O VER THE years I've learned that, to most people, *safe* and *toxic* are polar opposites: in their minds, a product is either completely all right to use or seriously harmful to health.

And many people think that all "toxic" products are toxic to the same degree. They think, for example, that food additives are as dangerous as pesticides because both are "toxic," when in fact pesticides are much more harmful.

Actually, the safety or toxicity of a product is not as absolute as simply being "safe" or "toxic." There are many variations and gradations of inherent toxicity among products, and a number of factors that can affect whether or not the product will cause harm to you individually.

When you learn how each toxic exposure can be different, you can easily assess the risk of different exposures you may encounter, and decide for yourself whether it's important to eliminate or reduce your exposure.

The entire field of toxicology exists to scientifically study poisons and their effects on human bodies and other living systems. While toxicology books are big and heavy and have a lot of words most of us don't understand, the basic concepts are actually pretty simple.

When you understand how poisons work in relation to your body, you can be your own toxicologist and figure out how to minimize the effects a toxic exposure may have on your own body.

Toxicologists do studies and find out if chemicals have health effects on the subjects of their studies. However, whether or not a particular toxic exposure will affect *your* body depends a great deal on the nature of the specific exposure you have.

Factors that can affect the harm that comes to you from exposure to a toxic substance are:

- the inherent toxicity of the substance
- what happens to the substance once it enters your body
- how often you are exposed to the substance
- the amount of the substance you are exposed to
- the amounts of toxic chemicals that are already stored in your body
- if you belong to a high-risk group

Let's take a look at each of these in more detail.

Inherent Toxicity

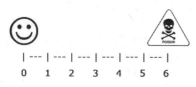

Toxicity rating
1 practically nontoxic
2 slightly toxic
3 moderately toxic
4 very toxic
5 extremely toxic
6 supertoxic

Probable lethal dose*
more than 1 quart
1 pint to 1 quart
1 ounce to 1 pint
1 teaspoon to 1 ounce
7 drops to 1 teaspoon
a taste (less than 7 drops)

* for 150-pound man

There is an inherent toxicity to each substance on earth.

The *toxicity* of a poison is the relative degree of harm that potentially could be caused by it. There is a whole gradient scale of toxicity from "Not at all toxic" to "A drop will kill you."

Toxicologists have developed a rating scale to compare

the potency of chemicals causing similar responses. It ranges from 1, for chemicals that are practically nontoxic, to 6, for chemicals that are supertoxic.

The numbers and associated terms related to specific doses are known as "LD50." If the biological response is death, the dose that kills 50 percent of the exposed population is known as the lethal dose 50, or LD50.

The dose that is used to establish these ratings is the LD50 for a 150-pound man. Of course, if you are considering the toxic dose for an infant or child or elderly person, or someone who is ill, the amount that would cause harm would be much less.

You can use these numbers and terms as guidelines to compare the toxicity of chemicals with each other. However, you cannot use them to compare how toxic they would be to various individuals. Age, sex, health condition, and more all contribute to how toxic a chemical is to an individual body.

Toxicokinetics: What Happens to Toxics in Your Body

Kinetics is the branch of biochemistry concerned with measuring and studying the rates of reactions.

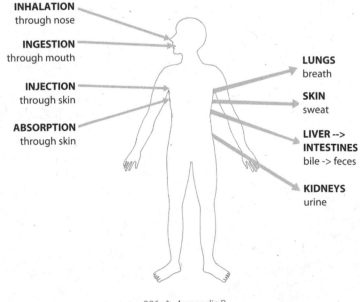

INHALATION
through nose

INGESTION
through mouth

INJECTION
through skin

ABSORPTION
through skin

LUNGS
breath

SKIN
sweat

**LIVER -->
INTESTINES**
bile -> feces

KIDNEYS
urine

Toxicokinetics, then, is the branch of toxicology concerned with measuring and studying the rates of reactions of toxic chemicals in a body (human, animal, or plant) or the environment (air, water, or soil). It is the description of how a chemical will enter a body and what happens to that chemical once it is inside that body.

Toxicokinetics are used in risk assessments to determine the potential effects of releasing chemicals into the environment where humans and other species would be exposed to them.

Toxicokinetics are also used to describe and predict the behavior of a toxicant in a body, including how the toxicant enters your body, what happens to the toxicant within your body, and how the toxicant might leave your body.

ROUTES OF ENTRY

There are four routes by which toxic substances can enter your body. Some chemicals are toxic regardless of how they enter the body; others, for example, can be toxic by ingestion but are safe to inhale. When toxic effects are given in toxicology books and databases, they give the toxic effects by various means of exposure.

Mouth

Ingestion—eating or drinking a substance—is how most immediate poisonings occur that lead to accidental death. Toxic substances that enter your body through your mouth can be absorbed through the lining of your mouth, stomach, and intestines, though most are absorbed in the small intestine.

If these linings are damaged by inflammation, ulcers, or infection, even more of the chemical is absorbed. Absorption is also affected by the type and amount of food in your stomach and intestines.

Toxic chemicals can also enter your body through your mouth by inhalation of toxics that are present in the air.

Nose

Toxic exposure by **inhalation**—breathing a substance—is more common, and can be much more harmful than ingestion. Often we are not aware of small inhalant exposures. Dusts, mists, and particulates can get stuck in your lungs, while gases are immediately absorbed.

In addition to irritating your nose, throat, and lungs, when you inhale toxic fumes, the poisons go directly into your bloodstream and quickly travel to organs like your brain, heart, liver, and kidneys.

The amount of chemical you receive through inhalation is affected by how often and how deeply you breathe, the condition of your lungs—asthmatics and others with lung conditions are more susceptible—and the concentration of the substance.

Toxic fumes can be released even when a chemical is tightly sealed in its container. If you doubt this, simply walk down the cleaning-products or pesticide aisle at your local supermarket and take a whiff. Notice how strongly it smells of toxic chemicals, even though all the containers are sealed tight.

Good ventilation in your home helps dilute airborne toxics and makes them less harmful.

Skin

Absorption—admitting a substance into the body through the skin—is often unsuspected as a route of exposure.

In times past, the skin was thought to be an impermeable, protective coating. We now know that any chemical that touches the skin can be absorbed and spread throughout the body. The skin is so absorbent that nicotine patches and analgesic creams now administer medications into the bloodstream through the skin.

Skin absorption is obvious when you apply a product, such as cream or lotion, to your skin, but can also occur unintentionally, such as when your hands are immersed in a cleaning solution. When skin is damaged by burns, cuts, and inflammation, chemicals can permeate even more easily.

Absorption rates vary for different body parts:

BODY PART	% ABSORBED
Forearm	9%
Palm of hand	12%
Scalp	32%
Ear canal	46%
Scrotum	100%

Toxics can also enter the body through the skin via injection. This is not a common route of exposure for household poisons. Generally, the only toxic substances that enter the body via injection are drugs.

Eyes

Any liquid chemical can easily be splashed in the eyes, but there are also other means of entry. Chemicals on hands can be rubbed in the eyes. Dust in the air can end up in the eyes. Aerosol sprays produce fine mists that can irritate the eyes.

ABSORBABILITY

Absorbability is how easy or difficult it is for the toxicant to be taken in by your body.

In order to harm a body, enough poison must:

- get into a body, and then
- be absorbed by that body

All poisons are matter in the state of solid, liquid, or gas. The larger the particle, the more difficult it is for the body to absorb.

Solids are difficult for the body to absorb. Particles of lead in its elemental form as found in the earth, for example, is practically nontoxic because it does not dissolve in water and therefore cannot be absorbed. The industrial chemical lead sulfate, however, is soluable in water and therefore can be absorbed.

Liquids are easy for the body to absorb. Liquid cleaning products and pesticides, for example, can be absorbed by the body quite readily.

Gases are very easy for the body to absorb. Gases include any chemicals that evaporate into the air, including vapors from plastics, fragrances, and especially aerosol sprays, which take liquids and make a mist that is very easy to absorb through lungs and skin.

SOLUBILITY

Solubility is whether or not a chemical can dissolve in water or fat. This is an important distinction that affects how a chemical moves through your body and the process your body uses to excrete it.

A chemical that can be dissolved in water is called water-soluble and a chemical that can be dissolved in fat is called fat-soluble. Whether a certain chemical is water-soluble or fat-soluble makes a big difference in how it is absorbed by your body.

In order for chemicals to get into your body, they have to pass through various membranes. These membranes are primarily composed of fatty material, so when fat-soluble molecules come in contact with a membrane, they simply dissolve into the membrane and come through on the other side. Because they can dissolve right through membranes, fat-soluble chemicals are difficult for your body to get rid of. Whenever a fat-soluble chemical is collected by your body and taken to a storage location (such as your liver, gallbladder, or small intestine) to await elimination, it dissolves right through the storage membranes and back into your bloodstream.

Water-soluble chemicals require a different method to get through membranes, known as direct transport, which evolved to move nutrients across membranes. Many toxic substances share a resemblance to nutrients, so they are able to fool the body and use this system to get through membrane barriers. The problem is, there are only "so many seats on the boat," so to speak, and if these are taken up by molecules of water-soluble chemicals, there is no room for the nutrients to be delivered to the cells.

DISTRIBUTION

Once a chemical is inside a body, it is distributed through the bloodstream to all the organs of the body. However, three processes prevent the potentially damaging chemical from hitting all the organs at the same time.

Metabolism

Metabolism begins almost immediately after the chemical enters your body. Metabolism has the ability to detoxify some chemicals by turning them into a less toxic form called a *metabolite*.

This sounds like a good thing, but what happens is that sometimes, harmless chemicals are *bioactivated* or made more harmful, by metabolic transformations. Often it is not known whether the original chemical or its bioactivated metabolite is causing the toxic reaction.

Ideally, chemicals that need to be bioactivated before causing harm should be eliminated from the body quickly, before the body has a chance to render them harmful. Unfortunately, your body's disposal service may be running slow.

Sometimes exposure to one chemical, even at nontoxic doses, can cause the body to bioactivate other chemicals and make them more harmful. This is known as *synergistic effects*. In my first book, *Nontoxic & Natural*, I wrote about a study done by Dr. Benjamin Ershoff and the Institute for Nutritional Studies in Culver City, California. Rats were given different combinations of three common food additives: sodium cyclamate, the food dye Red No. 2, and polyoxyethylene sorbitan monostearate (sorbitol). At first the rats were fed only one of the three additives, and nothing happened. Then, the test animals were given sodium cyclamate and Red No. 2; they stopped growing, lost their hair, and developed diarrhea. When the rats were finally given all three additives, they lost weight rapidly and all died within two weeks.

Binding to Blood Proteins

Many toxic chemicals are attracted to proteins in blood plasma and are capable of attaching to these proteins as they circulate in the bloodstream. This reduces the amount of the toxic chemical available to damage organs, but it also prolongs the time that a toxic substance circulates in the body. Bound toxic molecules cannot harm their target organ, but they can become unbound and later do their damage. This is what happens when the body has a time-delayed response rather than an immediate poisoning.

In most cases, this gives the body time to break down the chemical into a metabolite without being poisoned. But as I've already outlined above, this is not always what happens.

Storage in Body Tissue

Another way your body can prevent toxic chemicals from causing harm is by storing the chemicals in your body tissues, such as fat and bone. While most toxicants will not harm your body while sequestered away, large amounts of stored chemicals can be released into your bloodstream, sometimes years after the initial exposure, if the storage location is disturbed. If stored fat, for example, is metabolized during weight loss, the chemicals stored in that fat will be released into circulation. Likewise, during pregnancy, a woman's body may tap into calcium reserves in her bones, causing the lead that is stored there to be released as well. This may result in high levels of lead in the bloodstream of the mother and her unborn child.

EXCRETION

If the metabolites are not bound to proteins or stored in body tissue, they usually leave your body.

Some chemicals leave your body by the same route they came in. If you breathe in a toxic solvent from a permanent marker and exhale quickly, much of that solvent will come right back out before it can be absorbed into the bloodstream by the lungs. And ingested chemicals that are difficult to absorb will go right through the intestines and out with feces.

Otherwise, toxicants are excreted from the body through the kidneys, liver, and skin, which are described in greater detail in Chapter 4.

Frequency of Exposure

Remember the definition of *poisoning*. In order for a poisoning to occur, there needs to be enough poison in the body to cause injury. And frequency of exposure contributes to the amount of poison that gets into the body.

There are two aspects to frequency of exposure.

The first is obvious: how often you are exposed to the poison greatly affects how much of a poison ends up in your body. There is a big difference, for example, between being exposed to toxic fumes from pumping gas into your car once a week versus breathing gas fumes all day long every day.

The second has to do with single exposure versus ongoing everyday exposure.

Acute exposure refers to poisoning as the result of a onetime exposure to a relatively large amount of a chemical, such as a child accidentally drinking from a bottle of lemon-scented furniture polish. Acute toxicity is a concern for most consumer products that have warning labels, and is the reason we have poison control centers. Every year, five to ten million household poisonings are reported as the result of accidental exposure to toxic products in the home. Some are fatal, and most of the victims are children. These poisonings are the result of accidental ingestion of common household products that, despite warning labels, are not kept out of children's reach. Some of the most common acute exposures include medications, cleaning supplies, cosmetics and personal care products, plants, and pesticides.

Chronic exposure refers to illness as the result of many repeated exposures to small amounts of a chemical over a long period of time, such as cancer caused by smoking cigarettes. That a toxic effect can build up over time is what makes it so difficult to identify some toxics. We can easily see the effects when drain cleaner is spilled on someone's hand and the skin burns. The effects of chronic toxicity may not show up for years. Numerous common household products can cause cancer—not an immediate effect, because carcinogenic substances take twenty years or more to act. Other household chemicals are mutagenic: they can change genetic material and lead to health problems. Still others are known to be teratogenic, and the high incidence of birth defects continues to remind us that not all household substances have been tested for this danger.

Dose

Paracelsus, a Swiss Renaissance physician, botanist, alchemist, astrologer, and the father of toxicology, said, "All things are poison and nothing is without poison, only the dose permits something not to be poisonous." Or, more briefly: "The dose makes the poison."

Again, remember the definition of *poisoning*. For a poisoning to occur, there needs to be *enough* poison in your body to cause injury.

So you could be exposed to a small amount of a toxic substance and not have a toxic effect. If the toxicant goes right through your body, there would be no effect. But if you were (1) exposed to a large amount of a toxicant at one time or (2) exposed to many small amounts of a toxicant over time and they accumulated in your body, then the dose would be great enough to cause a symptom or illness. The more poison there is in your body, the greater the response. This is the case with all known poisons.

Dose is actually more important than the toxicity of a chemical. For example, *botulinum toxin* is not especially hazardous, even though it is supertoxic, because food is well-preserved, keeping the exposure or dose very low. In contrast, ethanol (alcohol) is hazardous even though it is not very toxic, because some people have a tendency to use it to excess.

You could have a glass of wine with dinner and it probably would not be a problem. You might, however, get drunk (a toxic response) if you drank the whole bottle. That's the importance of dose.

On the other hand, with some chemicals the poison isn't entirely in the dose. Research shows that endocrine disruptors, for example, can be "hand-me-down" poisons—parents exposed to the chemicals are fine, but their children suffer the toxic effects.

What makes this a little trickier is that the toxic dose varies from individual to individual. The same amount of a substance could have no effect on one individual and make another very sick.

High-Risk Groups

Some people are much more sensitive to toxic chemicals than others, and need to take greater precautions to minimize their exposure to toxicants.

PREGNANT WOMEN

Those most vulnerable to the toxic effects of exposure to chemicals in consumer products are the new lives growing in their mothers' wombs. So if you are pregnant, or plan to be pregnant, it is most important that you minimize as much as possible your own toxic exposures and remove toxic chemicals from your body, for whatever toxic chemicals you are exposed to sooner or later will find their way to the baby in your womb.

Toxic exposures that affect the health of your child in the womb, at birth, and even later in life begin even before you conceive your child. If you are like most women, you are exposed to toxic chemicals in amounts greater than your body can handle, so you now have a body burden of chemicals stored in your fat, bones, and other tissues that can later be released and transferred to your baby in your womb. Exposure to toxic chemicals can also make it difficult or impossible to conceive, and cause miscarriages.

Every toxic chemical you breathe, eat, or put on your skin while pregnant goes right into your bloodstream and is carried throughout your body, including right to your growing baby. Your yet-to-be-born child has no defenses in place to withstand these exposures. Today, sadly, this is simply a fact of life.

According to an article in *Environmental Health Perspectives*, an analysis of chemical exposure data from 268 pregnant women from the National Health and Nutrition Examination Survey revealed that certain PCBs, organochlorine pesticides, PFCs, phenols, PBDEs, phthalates, polycyclic aromatic hydrocarbons (PAHs), and perchlorate were detected in 99 to 100 percent of pregnant women. So it's very likely that your body contains these chemicals too.

And research shows that toxic chemicals are found in newborns as well. The Environmental Working Group tested the umbilical cord blood of ten minority babies and found as many as 232 chemicals in the ten newborns. Nine out of the ten tested positive for BPA, an industrial petrochemical that has been associated with cancer, cognitive and behavioral impairments, endocrine system disruption, reproductive and cardiovascular system abnormalities, diabetes, asthma, and obesity.

BABIES AND CHILDREN

Infants and children have greater risk for health effects from toxic exposures than adults, with infants having the greater risk.

The most direct risks to babies and children are toxic products around your home that can cause immediate poisoning. Because of their natural curiosity, young children are especially vulnerable to household poisonings through ingestion. Children learn by putting things in their mouths, and they cannot tell the difference between some toxic chemicals and things they think are good. It's easy for them to confuse lemon-scented toxic furniture polish with lemonade, for example, because they both smell the same. Ammonia looks like apple juice. Children don't know that the mothball designed to kill insects isn't candy when it has the same size and shape. And children can't read warning labels. Each year five to ten million accidental poisonings are reported to U.S. poison control centers. Many are fatal, and most of the victims are children.

Beyond immediate poisonings, children are at higher risk for the effects of long-term exposures to household toxicants as well.

To begin with, children's playing habits cause them to come in more direct contact with toxics. Indoors, children crawl around on carpets, rubbing their bodies on formaldehyde-based resins and breathing air close to the floor, where heavier pollutants settle. Outdoors, they roll around on the grass and climb trees, coming into contact with pesticides and other toxic hazards in the soil.

Infants and children come into greater contact with ingested toxicants than adults. They consume larger amounts of fruit juice and vegetables than are typically consumed by adults; these are common sources of exposure for pesticides unless they are organically grown. Children also drink two to five times more water than adults, giving them an increased ratio of body weight to water pollutants. And, once ingested, metals like lead and cadmium—both found in tap water—are absorbed more efficiently through the gastrointestinal tract of the young. Children up to age eight, for example, can absorb up to five times as much lead as adults, and they retain it longer.

Air pollutants also pose a greater risk to infants and children. Children require more oxygen, and they breathe in two to three times more air (and therefore more air pollutants) relative to body size than adults. Children are more physically active than adults, which also increases their breathing rate and intake of pollutants. And because children suffer more respiratory illness, their frequently blocked nasal passages make them breathe more often through their mouths, which doesn't filter out particles the way nose breathing does. Once ingested, toxic substances can injure lung tissue and be absorbed into the bloodstream.

The detoxification systems in your child's liver and kidneys that normally neutralize and excrete toxicants are not yet fully developed, and their immune system is not yet fully functional. Humans do not build up adult levels of antibodies until around ten years of age. So, in effect, your child is walking around in the world being bombarded with the same toxic exposure as you are as an adult, but without the natural protective armor that your body has.

The blood-brain barrier that protects the human brain from some toxic chemicals is not completely formed in the body of your infant, either. Once inside the brain, neurotoxicants can have devastating effects. Cells of the developing nervous system are actively growing, dividing, and migrating as well as forming complex networks. Neurotoxic chemicals can interfere with these steps, leading to permanent problems like learning disabilities.

It is especially important that newborns be protected from household toxics, for their bodily systems are the most vulnerable of all. Yet, this is the time when many parents—albeit with good intentions—create very toxic worlds for their babies to live in. A room often is redecorated into a nursery, with new paint, washable vinyl wallpaper with little animals, a new crib with a synthetic mattress and brand-new no-iron sheets, new easy-care synthetic clothing, disinfectants (especially disinfectants to protect the baby from germs), scented baby lotions and powders, stuffed animals made from synthetic fibers, plastic rattles . . . And as the child grows, there is more remodeling, more new plastic toys, more new synthetic clothes. I'm not saying here that children shouldn't have or don't need new things, but the constant newness of everything gives children more frequent exposure to toxicants than adults—who tend to use things for a longer period of time—would have.

The result of all these chemical exposures can be seen in the decline in our children's health. Asthma, once a very rare disease, is now common in children. Childhood asthma has increased by more than 40 percent since 1980, and according to the EPA, asthma deaths in children and young people increased by 118 percent between 1980 and 1993.

Illnesses that didn't even exist when I was a child are now common. Asthma, cancer, learning disabilities, attention deficit disorder, behavior disorders . . . Although other factors are involved, all of these illnesses and more have been associated with exposure to toxic chemicals.

Because the rise in the incidence of childhood diseases has been so dramatic, in November 1996 the EPA announced that for the first time children would be considered in all their risk-assessment and standard-setting procedures. In April 1997, President Clinton signed Executive Order No. 13045 (Protection of Children from Environmental Health Risks and Safety Risks), requiring federal agencies to include children and their unique susceptibilities when setting standards.

On many fronts now, whether or not a chemical exposure is safe for children is the primary question. And it should be. For what is safe for a child will be safe for an adult, whereas what may be safe for an adult often is not safe for a child.

WOMEN

Women tend to be more at risk than men to the effects of toxicants.

Women's bodies are generally smaller than the bodies of men, which means the amount of pollutants they are exposed to by comparison is greater in relation to their body weight. If a man and a woman are both living in the same household, the woman will be exposed to more pollution relative to her body weight than the man, thus giving her the greater exposure.

Women also have higher levels of hormones that are extremely vulnerable to certain toxicants. And women have more fat cells in which fat-soluble toxicants can accumulate; thus women can have a greater body burden.

THE ELDERLY

The elderly are also more at risk to the effects of toxic chemicals.

By the time a body has had sixty or seventy years or more of toxic exposure, it is likely to be full of stored toxic chemicals, if nothing has been done to remove them. This in and of itself can cause aging and premature death.

But also, all body systems are no longer functioning as efficiently, and detox systems are likely to be exhausted.

PEOPLE WITH CERTAIN GENETIC DEFECTS

How well your body can detoxify and eliminate chemicals depends on the presence of certain enzymes. Genetics determine which enzymes are available for your body's detoxification processes, and some people do not have enough specific detoxification enzymes, due to the genetic makeup of their bodies. These people are at higher risk to the health effects of toxic chemicals.

Geneticists theorize that as the population is exposed to more chemicals, more individuals with abnormal enzymes will be found.

As only one example, one of the enzymes that metabolizes drugs and chemicals is debrisoquine hydroxylase. It is controlled by a single gene that has different forms. Individuals with slow rates of debrisoquine hydroxylation are found more frequently in European populations. In several epidemiological studies, Parkinson's disease has been associated with pesticide use. Individuals who cannot metabolize and rid their bodies of pesticides because of faulty debrisoquine hydroxylase may then become more susceptible to Parkinson's disease.

PEOPLE WITH MULTIPLE CHEMICAL SENSITIVITIES

Multiple chemical sensitivity (MCS) is a condition involving intolerance of certain chemicals found in the everyday environment. They are the result of a specific malfunction of the immune system. To me, this is the ultimate chemical insult, because with MCS, toxic chemicals cause damage to your immune system, making you sensitive to that chemical and many others. Life then becomes a series of one toxic chemical reaction after another.

In 1982, I coauthored an article, "Multiple Chemical Sensitivities and Immune System Dysregulation," with immunologist Alan S. Levin, M.D. This is how we described the illness then:

> For someone with this immune malfunction, a substance can provoke any one or more of a number of symptoms, including traditional "allergic" nasal stuffiness, wheezing, sneezing, asthma, chronic sore throat, postnasal drip, laryngitis, itching eyes, hives, and rashes. In addition, gastrointestinal disturbances such as gastric irritation, bloating, intermittent constipation or diarrhea, hemorrhoids, or anal bleeding may occur. Musculoskeletal aches, pains, or twitching, and arthritis or rheumatism are some other common reactions, as well as problems in a host of other body systems, such as frequent or painful urination, menstrual cramps, body or breath odors, metallic aftertaste, sensitivity to light, visual disturbances, and ringing in the ears.

The most surprising and dramatic documented environmentally-induced symptoms by far are the cerebral and behavioral reactions. These include migraine headaches, fatigue, dizziness, learning disabilities, confusion, inability to concentrate, lack of motivation, memory loss, and dyslexia. Personality changes, mood swings, hyperactivity and depression are also common.

In addition, another common behavioral symptom is insatiable hunger, leading to incessant eating and often to obesity. Addictions to specific foods, such as wheat, corn, sugar, coffee, and chocolate can also develop, as well as addictions to alcoholic beverages, drugs, tobacco, and even some common chemical vapors, such as perfume, hairspray, or glue. . . .

In addition, immune system dysregulation reduces the immune system's ability to fight infection, leaving the body vulnerable to various illnesses caused by bacteria, viruses, and fungi.

These were our clinical observations then, based on what we were seeing in the patients that came to his office in 1982. Neurological symptoms are not surprising: it's now well known that neurotoxicants can cause these symptoms with or without immune system malfunctions.

Of course, individuals with such an immune malfunction need to be extremely cautious about their exposure to chemical toxicants.

APPENDIX C

Risk Management

THOUGH WE LIVE in a world full of toxic exposures, there is much each of us can do to minimize loss. The whole field of *risk management* is about taking action to minimize loss, and these tried-and-true strategies can be easily applied to minimizing the loss of health associated with toxic chemical exposures.

Here are the basic concepts behind risk management.

A *hazard* is something that has the potential to cause harm or loss. Bungee jumping is a hazard. Playing golf on a golf course in a lightning storm is a hazard. Using an electric hairdryer in the bathtub is a hazard. And toxic chemical exposure is a hazard.

If you know something is a hazard and know the likely loss that would result from doing it, then you can do something to eliminate or lessen the loss.

This entire book is about managing the risk of loss from exposure to toxic chemicals.

To take a *risk* is to participate in the hazard—to put yourself in harm's way—thereby creating a probability that harm or loss could happen.

Risk is determined by multiplying the expected consequences by the rate of occurrence. Here in Florida, where I live, for example, we have alligators in the water. This is definitely a hazard, because if you go in the water with alligators, there is a high probability the alligators will attack your body. But here's the important thing to grasp: *An alligator in the water is not a risk until you put your body in or near the water.* Likewise, a toxic chemical is not a risk until you put your body next to it, or put it next to or on or in your body.

With regard to toxic chemicals, risk is determined by multiplying the expected health effects to your own body by the frequency with which you are exposed to the toxic chemical.

You can reduce the risk to your health by:

- reducing your exposures to toxic chemicals in your home and the environment (thereby reducing the frequency of exposure)
- increasing your body's ability to process and eliminate the toxic chemicals it is exposed to (thereby reducing expected health effects)

There is a standard protocol for risk management that serves well to manage the risk of exposure to toxic chemicals:

Identify Hazards and Their Expected Consequences

The key to risk management is to be aware of that which can cause harm to you.

Identification of many toxic chemicals that cause specific health and environmental hazards has already been done, and new studies are continuously being done that identify more threats.

Two major toxic threats that are already identified and have risk management in place are cigarettes and alcohol. Warnings have been widely issued regarding both and they are considered risk factors for likelihood of disease and reduced life expectancy.

Toxic chemicals in consumer products likewise need to be considered risk factors for the likelihood of disease and reduced life expectancy.

While researching risk management, I went to a website that assessed your risk for certain diseases and life expectancy. A number of factors were considered, including smoking and drinking, but there was not one question regarding toxic chemical exposure. Yet, we are exposed daily to toxic chemicals that are contributing to our risk of developing life-threatening illness and which reduce our life expectancy.

Access the Vulnerability of Specific Assets to the Hazards

With toxic chemicals, the critical assets are your body and the environment that supports your life (without the environment, your body would have no air, water, food, or other natural resources that contribute to your body being alive and healthy).

The vulnerability of the health of your body depends on the condition of your body and its ability to withstand exposure to the toxic chemicals it is exposed to. This varies from body to body.

Manage Risk by Considering Ways to Reduce It

There are four general strategies that can be used to reduce risk.

AVOIDANCE

Avoidance is about eliminating, withdrawing from, and not becoming involved with a risk. With regard to toxic chemical exposure, that would simply be to eliminate toxic chemicals in your immediate environment, both at home and at work.

In the world of risk management, avoidance may not be the best solution for all risk because some benefits might also be eliminated; however, in most cases toxics can be completely eliminated, and benefits can still be had, by replacing the toxic product with a toxic-free product that has the same benefit. Toxic-free cleaning products, for example, clean just fine without the toxic risk. Organically grown food tastes even better and has more nutrition, without the risk of pesticide exposure found in nonorganic foods.

In more than thirty years of living toxic-free, in almost every case I have been able to find a nontoxic alternative to every toxic exposure.

REDUCTION

Avoidance is the number one preferred strategy to apply, but if that isn't possible for whatever reason, there are two ways to reduce the risk if you must be exposed to a toxic chemical. Reduce the likelihood of the loss occurring:

- **Keep toxics out of reach of children.**
- **Keep products in their original containers so the original label is available in case of accidental poisoning and to prevent confusion.** Accidental poisoning often occurs when look-alike poisons are stored in food and drink containers.
- **Use only the amount of a product that the directions call for.** Using more hardly ever makes a product more effective and can make the exposure more harmful.
- **Keep containers tightly closed to prevent volatile fumes from escaping.**
- **Use products in a well-ventilated area to dilute the fumes.** Use the product outdoors, if possible. If you must use the product indoors, open windows, turn on a stove hood or ventilation fan, or use air-to-air exchangers.
- **Don't mix chemicals.** Some combinations, such as chlorine bleach and ammonia (or products such as scouring powders and all-purpose cleaners, which contain these substances), can produce toxic fumes. If you are not a chemist, you don't know what you'll end up with.
- **Shield your body from the exposure with protective gear such as masks, gloves, or even a hazmat suit if the occasion warrants it.** Particularly wear protective clothing if it is recommended on the label.
- **Buy only what you need and use it up, or dispose of it properly.**
- **Carefully clean up after using toxics.** Make sure products are properly stored, spills are wiped up, and rags are properly disposed of.

- **Use air or water filters to reduce the amount of toxic exposure.**
- **Use the product only occasionally.**

These precautions will reduce your own risk of health effects, but the manufacture and disposal of the product may still have environment effects, and can come back to you indirectly through an environmental exposure.

Reduce the severity of the loss by improving the ability of your body to withstand exposure without consequences.

SHARING

To share the risk usually means to outsource the risk or to insure against loss. That's what insurance is about: having someone else share the loss, should it occur, whether the loss is your house burning down or a car accident or catastrophic health problems.

With toxic chemicals, you can outsource exposures by having someone else do the activity that results in the exposure. You could, for example, have someone else paint your house so you would not be exposed to the toxic fumes during application of the paint.

Currently, you can't buy insurance to help defray the costs of health problems caused by exposures to toxic chemicals in consumer products. But it is my opinion that insurance companies should become aware of the risks and losses associated with toxic chemicals in our daily lives and incorporate toxic chemicals as a risk factor in their programs. For example, an insurance company could lower premiums for customers who live in toxic-free homes, similar to reduced premiums for nonsmokers. If insurance companies were to educate customers on how to lessen their toxic exposures, they could save a lot of money paying on health insurance claims. For toxic chemicals are causing illness, whether or not they are recognized as the cause.

RETENTION

Retention is to accept the risk and budget resources to handle the consequences when they occur.

With regard to toxic chemical exposure, this would be to continue to be exposed to toxic chemicals, do nothing to improve your body's ability to process and eliminate toxic chemicals, and budget for the cost of illnesses that result.

To me, this strategy is entirely unnecessary, as much can be done to avoid, reduce, and share the risk.

PRIORITIZE RISK REDUCTION MEASURES BASED ON A STRATEGY

After you identify risk reduction measures, the next step is to prioritize them.

For toxic chemicals, this would be to determine which steps are most important to take first, and that will reduce risk the most.

Generally, this would be to take measures to eliminate or reduce your greatest exposures to the most toxic chemicals in your home.

PLAN TO IMPLEMENT RISK REDUCTIONS

Finally, make a plan as to how you are going to take the actions needed to reduce the exposures.

Precautionary Principle

Whenever you are in doubt, the best bet is to apply the *precautionary principle.*

The precautionary principle is about making decisions that are most likely to result in supporting life. It basically suggests that if an action is suspected to cause harm to health or the environment, it's better to err on the side of caution.

This is an old concept, captured in many traditional aphorisms: "An ounce of prevention is worth a pound of cure," "Better safe than sorry," "Look before you leap."

The precautionary principle also includes the concept of "preventative anticipation," which is a willingness to take action in advance of scientific proof of evidence if there is reason to believe the action would be harmful to health or the environment.

This has been my personal philosophy since the beginning of my work with household toxics, and over the years, many of my precautionary recommendations have been later proven by science.

/

How to Determine If a Product Is Toxic

T WOULD BE NICE if every safe product had a little sticker on it that said SAFE, but they don't. And I'm not even sure they could. I think if you were to ask a manufacturer, an industry spokesperson, a government regulator, an average consumer, and me if a specific product is safe, you would get five different answers. And because of your own individual degree of tolerance, personal taste, and budget, only you can decide how to choose safe products that are right for you.

Determining the toxicity of any product can be difficult because there are so many factors to consider. It's easy to identify some substances that are inherently unsafe, such as the bacteria that cause botulism, or benzene, which has known harmful effects; but tracking down the toxicity of other substances can be a much more complex process.

Toxicity of a substance is scientifically determined primarily through the use of animal studies in controlled laboratory experiments, although studies are sometimes made on human subjects if the effect of the substance is thought to be reversible. An experiment to find acute effects (known as the LD_{50}) determines the dose that causes the immediate death of 50 percent of the animals. Experiments on chronic effects might look for changes in blood chemistry, enzyme activity, tissue damage, and cancer induction over a period of a few months or even years. Some experiments require several generations of animals. Though animal rights activists may object, the government requires these animal tests by law to assess the potential hazards of compounds before they are released for use by the general population.

Epidemiological studies are also used. They show a statistical correlation between the occurrence of disease in a population and the factors suspected of causing that disease. These studies often begin with a clinical observation, such as an unusually high frequency of cancer among those who smoke. They are valuable because they are based on the actual occurrences of real diseases in humans.

To determine if a particular product is harmful or safe for *you* to use, follow these steps.

Look for and Read the Warning Label on the Product.

Throughout this book, you will find examples of warning labels found on various products, such as cleaning products, pesticides, and paints. But warning labels are not required on all types of products, so don't assume that if there is no warning label, the product is safe. Some products containing formaldehyde, for example, require warning labels and others do not, even though the same formaldehyde is present in the product.

There is a legal definition of "toxic." According to Part 1500 of the 1960 Federal Hazardous Substances Act:

"Toxic" shall apply to any substance (other than a radioactive substance) which has the capacity to produce personal injury or illness to man through ingestion, inhalation, or absorption through any body surface. "Highly toxic" means any substance which falls within any of the following categories:

- Produces death within 14 days in half or more than half of a group of 10 or more laboratory white rats each weighing between 200 and 300 grams, at a single dose of 50 milligrams or less per kilogram of body weight, when orally administered; or

- Produces death within 14 days in half or more than half of a group of 10 or more laboratory white rats each weighing between 200 and 300 grams, when inhaled continuously for a period of 1 hour or less at an atmospheric concentration of 200 parts per million by volume or less of gas or vapor or 2 milligrams per liter by volume or less of mist or dust, provided such concentration is likely to be encountered by man when the substance is used in any reasonably foreseeable manner; or

- Produces death within 14 days in half or more than half of a group of 10 or more rabbits tested in a dosage of 200 milligrams or less per kilogram of body weight, when administered by continuous contact with the bare skin for 24 hours or less.

Later in the document, the Hazardous Substances Act notes that "highly toxic" also could refer to "a substance determined by the [Consumer Product Safety Commission] to be highly toxic on the basis of human experience." Based on these animal tests, the EPA has defined four categories of immediate acute toxicity that correspond to different dose levels received through ingestion, inhalation, and skin contact (see chart on page 231).

At one time, these signal words accurately indicated the dose required to cause a toxic effect; but because of poor labeling practices, these words now suggest only a general degree of danger.

While I was writing this book, I found it interesting to compare the label warnings with the actual dangers of the products, especially after my local poison control center had told me that about 85 percent of household items on the market are mislabeled! Some products are labeled as poison but really aren't; some are poisons but not labeled as such; some labels warn of dangers but don't list the poison; and many contain incorrect first-aid information.

SIGNAL WORDS FOR TOXIC PRODUCTS

CATEGORY	SIGNAL WORD(S)	APPROXIMATE AMOUNT NEEDED TO KILL AN AVERAGE PERSON	PRECAUTIONARY STATEMENT	
			ORAL, INHALATION, OR DERMAL TOXICITY	SKIN AND EYE LOCAL EFFECTS
I. Highly toxic	DANGER POISON	A few drops to 1 teaspoon	Fatal if swallowed (inhaled or absorbed through skin). Do not breathe vapor (dust or spray mist). Do not get in eye, on skin, or on clothing. (Front panel statement of treatment required.)	Corrosive, causes eye and skin damage (or skin irritation). Do not get in eyes, on skin, or clothing. Wear goggles or face shield and rubber gloves when handling. Harmful or fatal if swallowed. (Appropriate first-aid statement required.)
II. Moderately toxic	WARNING	1 teaspoon to 1 ounce	May be fatal if swallowed (inhaled or absorbed through skin). Do not breathe vapor (dust or spray mist). Do not get in eye, on skin, or on clothing. (Appropriate first-aid statement required.)	Causes eye and skin irritation. Do not get in eyes, on skin, or on clothing. Harmful if swallowed. (Appropriate first-aid statement required.)
III. Slightly toxic	CAUTION	More than 1 ounce	Harmful if swallowed (inhaled or absorbed through skin). Avoid breathing vapors (dust or spray mist). Avoid cotact with skin, eyes, or on clothing. (Appropriate first-aid statement required.)	Avoid contact with skin, eyes, or clothing. In case of contact, immediately flush eyes or skin with plenty of water. Get medical attention if irritation persists.
IV. Not toxic or nontoxic	(none required)		(none required)	(none required)

Also, label warnings are required only on products that are harmful or fatal if accidentally swallowed or inhaled in extreme concentrations. No warnings are given on products that affect health when used day in and day out over a long period of time. In many cases these effects are suspected but currently unknown.

If the warning label says DANGER: POISON, it is definitely toxic—do not use the product.

If the warning label says WARNING or CAUTION, it is acceptable.

Because these labels are used inconsistently, I do use some products with the WARNING or CAUTION label. Some of the least toxic products on the market have a CAUTION on the label because they are a powder, for example, and they need to warn that it is a possible eye irritant. If you use your common sense, you will be able to sort out which are the safe products.

To indicate long-term chronic hazards, the EPA has a classification scheme for cancer-causing agents, based on animal tests and epidemiological studies. Based on an assessment of the weight of evidence, these classifications are similar to those developed by the World Health Organization and the International Agency for Research on Cancer. Classification of a substance may change as new evidence, improved testing methods, or better analytical techniques become available, which also may affect regulations.

How to Read a Material Safety Data Sheet (MSDS)

Oa product that does not list ingredients—or for any product or chemical—is to get the material safety data sheet (MSDS) for the product.

An MSDS is designed to provide both workers and emergency personnel with the proper procedures for handling or working with toxic substances. They are required by the U.S. Occupational Health and Safety Administration (OSHA), a federal government agency within the U.S. Department of Labor, whose primary goals are to save lives, prevent injuries, and protect the health of America's workers.

Sometimes the information on an MSDS can be very revealing. I once requested the MSDS on a well-known cleaning product that advertises itself as nontoxic, socially responsible, and otherwise committed to the environment, and found glycol ether as the main ingredient. After I couldn't find this in my chemical dictionary, I called the manufacturer and was told that glycol ether was a class of substances and the specific glycol ether used was Butyl Cellosolve. This I did find in my dictionary as ethylene glycol monobutyl ether, a chemical so toxic that a major chemical company decided no longer to manufacture it. Butyl Cellosolve is neurotoxic and rapidly penetrates the skin. Once they diluted it down to 2 percent (98 percent of the product's plastic bottle is filled with water), the toxicity studies came out relatively harmless, but I had to ask myself if a product made from a diluted toxic chemical ethically should be called nontoxic. Not surprisingly, in 1994, a front-page story in my local newspaper reported that this company was being sued for misrepresentation of environmental claims.

It used to be that you had to contact the manufacturer to get a MSDS, but now most manufacturers post them on their websites. An easy way to find the MSDS for a product is to simply type "[brand name of product] MSDS" into your favorite search engine.

There are also more than 100 free Internet databases where you can look up the MSDSs for everything from single chemicals to generic and brand-name products. They are listed at www.ilpi.com/msds. This site also has an extremely useful glossary of abbreviations and terms used on MSDSs at www.ilpi.com/msds/ref/index.html.

An MSDS lists the ingredients, the manufacturer, hazards to safety and health, and precautions to follow when using the product. The sections are very straightforward and it is easy to read.

MSDSs are good for evaluating which products are toxic, but not very useful for identifying which products are safe. This is because manufacturers are required to report hazardous ingredients present only in concentrations greater than 1 percent, or 0.1 of 1 percent for carcinogens. Thus they are not a complete listing of ingredients or even a complete listing of hazardous ingredients. In addition, they do not list ingredients that you might consider to be toxic but which are not on official government lists of toxic ingredients. So use an MSDS to eliminate products with hazardous ingredients, but don't rely on them to verify that a product is safe.

MSDSs are easy to read. While the format of MSDSs varies, usually the same basic kinds of information is conveyed. Look for the following sections on the MSDS that will help you decide if the product is safe for you to use.

Hazardous Material Information System of the National Fire Protection Association

The quickest way to find out the toxicity of a product is to look for the health rating from the Hazardous Material Information System (HMIS; www.paint.org/hmis/index.cfm) or the National Fire Protection Association (NFPA; www.nfpa.org). These are two different rating systems that appear to be very similar, but they are not the same.

HMIS was developed by the American Coatings Association. It uses colored bars, numbers, and symbols to convey hazards. A label might look like this:

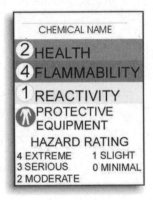

The NFPA uses colored diamonds. A label might look like this:

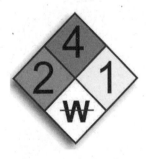

At first glance, these two systems seem to be very similar.

Both have four sections, which are color coded. You just need to look for the blue health section.

HMIS rating numbers in the blue bars indicate the following:

- 4—severe hazard
- 3—serious hazard
- 2—moderate hazard
- 1—slight hazard
- 0—minimal hazard

NFPA rating numbers in the blue diamond indicate the following:

- 4—Very short exposure could cause death or serious residual injury even though prompt medical attention was given.
- 3—Short exposure could cause serious temporary or residual injury even though prompt medical attention was given.
- 2—Intense or continued exposure could cause temporary incapacitation or possible residual injury unless prompt medical attention is given.
- 1—Exposure could cause irritation but only minor residual injury even if no treatment is given.
- 0—Exposure under fire conditions would offer no hazard beyond that of ordinary combustible materials.

The main difference is that the HMIS attempts to convey full health warning information for employees while the NFPA is meant primarily for firefighters and other emergency responders. The HMIS is not intended for emergency circumstances. Since you are simply evaluating the toxicity of a product or chemical so you can decide how you want to manage the risk, you can look at the blue health rating of either system.

CHEMICAL PRODUCT

This section lists the name of the product or chemical and the manufacturer.

If it is an MSDS for a single chemical, the CAS number will be given here (see page 15 for explanation of CAS number).

COMPOSITION / INFORMATION ON INGREDIENTS

This section lists the hazardous and/or regulated components in descending order according to the percentage amount contained in the product. Here you can see if a product contains a lot of a particular toxic chemical, or only a small amount.

Included here are the CAS numbers for each individual hazardous ingredient so you can do further research on each one if you want to.

This section also contains any hazard disclosures required.

HAZARDS IDENTIFICATION

This is the most important section because it contains the information on the health effects associated with using this product or chemical. It contains the major health hazards and potential health effects, which include the effects of short-term exposure through inhalation, skin contact, eye contact, and ingestion, the effects of long-term exposure, and the capacity for the substance to cause cancer.

FIRST-AID MEASURES

This section will give you more clues as to the toxicity of the product because it tells what to do in case you are exposed to this substance. If it says something like "take a ½ hour shower if you get the product on your skin" you'll know it's toxic.

ACCIDENTAL RELEASE MEASURES

This section gives instructions on what to do if there is an accidental spill. If it says something like "evacuate unprotected personnel from the area," you don't want to use this product or chemical at home.

HANDLING AND STORAGE

Look for the handling instructions here. The product is toxic if it says anything like "Avoid contact with eyes, skin, and clothing. Use with adequate ventilation. Do not swallow. Avoid breathing vapors, mists, or dust. Do not eat, drink, or smoke in work area. Wash thoroughly after handling."

EXPOSURE CONTROLS / PERSONAL PROTECTION

This section gives information about the ventilation system required, if personal respirators are needed, respiratory protection, skin protection, eye protection, and good hygiene conditions when working with this product or chemical. Obviously, if any are needed, the product is toxic.

TOXICOLOGICAL INFORMATION

Be sure to look for this section for the health effects of the product.

Here you will find the amount of each ingredient required to create a toxic effect when exposure occurs by ingestion, inhalation, or through the skin. Also, if the product has carcinogenic (causes cancer), mutagenic (damages genes), teratogenic (causes birth defects), or other toxic effects on humans.

ECOLOGICAL INFORMATION

This section explains how toxic the product is to the environment. You will generally find the following information (you may often encounter "not available"):

Ecotoxicity. This may contain data on specific species that are at risk, such as fish or birds.

BOD5 and COD. These are two of the most common generic indices used to assess aquatic organic pollution.

BOD5 is *biological oxygen demand*, which is used to evaluate how biodegradable or persistent the chemical is.

COD is *chemical oxygen demand*, which is the total organic pollution load of waters contaminated by reductive pollutants. Industries must continuously monitor COD to comply with regulatory requirements.

Products of Biodegradation. This tells the probability of hazardous chemicals resulting from biodegradation of the product or chemical, in the short and long term.

Toxicity of the Products of Biodegradation. This tells how toxic those products of biodegradation may be.

Special Remarks on the Products of Biodegradation. This usually tells the details of what happens when the product or chemical biodegrades.

DISPOSAL CONSIDERATIONS

If this section says the product needs to be disposed of as hazardous waste, it's not good for your health.

REGULATORY INFORMATION

This section shows which regulations govern these chemicals in different parts of the world.

Recommended Resources

FORTUNATELY, FAR too much information now exists on the safe alternatives to household toxics to be covered in one book. My intention in this guide has been to give you an overview of the subject and some first steps you can take.

Rather than adding extra pages to make lists of resources that will soon go out of date, I have put the recommended resources you would usually find in the back of a book on my website. There you will find:

Toxics & Health (www.toxics-health.com): more information on how toxic chemical exposures can affect your health.

Debra's List (www.debraslist.com): links to hundreds of sites that sell the safe and natural products mentioned in this book.

Debra's Bookstore (www.debrasbookstore.com): recommended books on toxics and safe alternatives, which you can purchase with a click.

Know Toxics Now (www.knowtoxicsnow.com): the data you need to make decisions about toxic-free products, including toxicity of ingredients and how to choose toxic-free products.

Toxic-Free Kitchen (www.toxicfreekitchen.com): my favorite recipes for preparing delicious toxic-free foods from fresh organic ingredients.

Debra Detox (www.debradetox.com): information about how to remove toxic chemicals from your body plus tips on choosing cookware, dinnerware, and more.

Personal Consultations (www.debralynndadd.com/consultations): I am available to answer your questions regarding toxic exposures and toxic-free products by phone, or on-site at your home or workplace.

I encourage you to make your own decisions after you do your own research and evaluations. Each author, editor, and organization holds a different perspective, and only you can decide what is right for you.

I would love to hear from you! Please e-mail me with your comments.
debra@dld123.com

Index

water, 64–65, 121–22
See also Indoor air pollution
Polybrominated diphenyl ethers, 19
Polychlorinated biphenyls (PCBs), 17, 116, 165, 169, 182, 215
Polyester, 93, 94, 96, 99, 102
Polypropylene, 93
Polyurethane, 96, 99, 102
Polyvinyl chloride (PVC), 92, 96, 97, 102
Polyvinylpyrrolidone (PVP), 69, 71
Porcelain enamel-coated cookware, 91
Prebiotics, 151
Precautionary principle, 227–28
Pregnancy, risk of toxics during, 215–16
Prescription drugs, 31, 32, 36
Probiotics, 149–51, 162
Protein, 146–48, 168
Public health, 127–28
Public transportation, 125
Purification Rundown, 169
Pyrethrin, 63

Radical Medicine (Williams), 6
Radioactive metals, 171
Recreational drugs, 31, 32
Recycled products, purchasing, 124
Recycling symbols, 44
Renewable energy, 124
Reproductive glands, 202
Resins, 19, 98–101. *See also* Formaldehyde
Respiratory system, 199–201
Right-to-Know Network, 120
Risk management, 222–28
Rubber cement, 109

Saccharin, 84
Safer Chemicals, Healthy Families coalition, 5
Salmonella, 51
Salt, 11, 12, 80, 85, 145, 157, 159, 202
San Francisco Household Hazardous Waste Program, 35
Saunas, 141, 162, 168–70
Scorecard, 20
Secondhand goods, purchasing, 124
Secondhand smoke, 27
Selden, Gary, 88–89
Sexy Forever (Somers), 7

Shampoo, 68–70, 72
lice, 63–64
Sheffield, University of, Center for Human Nutrition, 156
Shipping, global, 126
Shoes, 96–97
leaving at door, 37–38
Shower filters, 64–65
Silent Spring (Carson), 111–13
Silicone, 54
Silver, 145
Sinatra, Stephen T., 155
Skeletal system, 181–83
Skin, 134, 137, 140–41, 158, 185–86
strengthening, 162–63
absorption of toxics through, 208–9
Skin Deep, 67
Smoke, 11. *See also* Cigarettes
Soap, 24, 51, 68, 76–78
cleaning and laundry, 45, 48, 52, 56
tooth, 72
Soapnuts, 56
Sodium carbonate, 57
Sodium chloride, 11, 12, 145
Sodium hydroxide. *See* Lye
Sodium lauryl sulfate (SLS), 72
Soil, pollutants in, 112
Solar power, 124
Solubility, 210–11
Solvents, 24, 39, 108–9, 144, 181, 185, 186, 194, 195, 197, 199, 212
dry cleaning, 52–54
in home office products, 108, 109
in nail polish, 73, 74
in paints, 98–100
Somers, Suzanne, 7
Spot removers, 52
Stainless steel cookware, 90
Static cling, 57, 93
Steam, breathing, 163
Stevia, 87
Styrene, 17, 82, 104
Sucralose, 85
Sugar, 33, 80, 82, 84–88, 150
Sulfites, 31, 80, 88
Sulfur dioxide, 11, 125
Super Glue, 109
Supplements, 88–89, 148–53
Sweat, 140–41, 158, 162, 168–70